SIMPLE
CLEANSE

THE WEEKEND CLEANSE
AND
INTESTINAL HEALTH

Jerry Hutchens

Healthy Living Publications
Summertown, Tennessee

© 2005 by Jerry Lee Hutchens
Cover design by Warren Jefferson
Interior design by Jerry Lee Hutchens and Gwynelle Dismukes
Illustrations on pages 116 and 121 by Faith Hutchens
All other illustrations by the author

Published in the United States by
Healthy Living Publications
PO Box 99
Summertown, TN 38483
1 (888) 260-8458
www.bookpubco.com

07 06 05   3 2 1

ISBN: 1-57067-186-9

Library of Congress Cataloging-in-Publication Data

Hutchens, Jerry Lee.
  Simple cleanse : the weekend cleanse and intestinal health / Jerry Hutchens.
     p. cm.
  Includes bibliographical references and index.
  ISBN 1-57067-186-9
  1. Digestive organs--Diseases--Prevention--Popular works. 2. Digestive organs--
Diseases--Alternative treatment--Popular works. 3. Self-care, Health. I. Title.
  RC806.H88 2005
  616.3'06--dc22
                          2005018228

The information presented in this book is educational in nature and is not intended as medical advice. None of the statements made on these pages has been evaluated by any applicable government regulatory agency. This book is not intended to diagnose, treat, cure, or prevent any disease. The information presented here is as research and opinion only and is not conclusive. Always consult an appropriate health care practitioner before undertaking any kind of cleanse or medical treatment.

*This book is dedicated to those who will take control of
their health and go on to serve others.*

A heartfelt thanks to my dear wife, Kathryn,
for her support, insight, and sense of humor.
Thank you to Grandma Jessie Hutchens. Her understanding of
cleanliness continues to influence an expanding family.
To the health care professionals and lay people who reviewed and
commented on this work—you have my gratitude.

Contents

List of Illustrations

INTRODUCTION
to Simple Cleansing

We live in an environment filled with toxins and pollutants. This causes contaminants to enter our body and become lodged throughout our tissues. The systems our bodies have evolved for detoxifying and passing poisons strain under accumulations of toxic waste. We are burdened with artificial colorings, pesticide and herbicide residues, preservatives, and rancid oils in our foods. We are unable to escape from dangerous, chemical-based cleaning products and cosmetics, out-gassing particleboards, harmful medications, and a host of other insidious poisons. This bombardment is unrelenting. Poor eating habits and lack of exercise have further clogged our system, thwarting our body's natural ability to cleanse itself and eliminate the waste products of digestion and cell renewal.

If the external toxins we acquire from our environment and the internal toxins we naturally produce can be eliminated in a timely manner, our health will be maintained. However, the over-accumulation of waste products and toxins in our cells, tissues, and organs interferes with the nourishment and oxygenation of these tissues, leaving the body weak and susceptible to disease. This chronic excess of toxins negatively impacts our health and robs us of vitality, clear thinking, and the

THE SIMPLE CLEANSE PLAN

Nutrition	Exercise	Support Network	Weekend Cleanse
organic nutrient-packed high fiber plant-based	aerobic yogic stretching	loved ones health professionals others in similar situations	controlled two-day fast

robust life that is our potential. Therefore it is important that environmental toxins and cell wastes are eliminated from the body as quickly and efficiently as possible.

Despite all the unavoidable contaminants we are exposed to, there is a way to take control of our health. The answers offered in *Simple Cleanse* encompass healthful food, exercise, the Weekend Cleanse, and a support network of loved ones and health care professionals to share in the healing journey. I came to these solutions through trial and error, intense research, and a powerful desire to heal myself and to help others. Please understand that my intention with this book is to provide valuable information. This is not a substitute for medical attention.

Cleansing boosts our health by cleaning out the digestive tract, clearing tissues of toxic substances, increasing circulation, eliminating toxin-producing foods, and creating a healthful life. *Simple Cleanse* examines the marvelous way the body digests food, cleans the blood, and renews the cells. *Simple Cleanse* also reviews some of the typical ways these systems break down. The body has a wonderful capacity to heal and maintain good health, if we treat it right.

Cleansing gets the body in sync with its natural rhythms and cycles, ultimately allowing it to take care of itself. The path each person takes to this state of excellent health is unique. *Simple Cleanse* explains specific techniques for cleaning the digestive tract. Fasting, exercise, colon care, and diet are presented in detail. Here the word "diet" is used to talk about what and how we eat for optimum health, rather than its common interpretation as a temporary weight-loss regimen. To enjoy good health, we need to understand our current state of health, know our options, and begin the healing journey.

Toxins Everywhere

A mind-boggling number and variety of symptoms can be triggered by toxic overload. Pesticides can cause disruptions in both the nervous system and the endocrine system, as well as suppress the immune system. They are a pervasive source of carcinogens. Accumulated bowel toxicity has led naturopathic doctors to trace over 70 ailments to toxic bowels, including difficult to quantify symptoms such as bad dreams, "unclean" thoughts, fatigue, bloating, heart arrhythmia, diarrhea, constipation, fallen arches, tumors, high blood pressure, low blood pressure, drowsiness, insomnia, and appendicitis.[1] Evidence links industrial pollutants to lowered sperm counts.[2] Toxins gather in the blood and inside the ovaries.[3] Crossing the placental barrier, toxins negatively impact the fetus.[4] They are also slipped to our babies through breast milk.[5]

The worst of the synthetic chemicals found in pesticides, herbicides, building materials, and industrial wastes are collectively referred to as persistent organic pollutants (POPs). They are potent causes of cancer and are poisonous to the nervous system.[6] Before the early part of the 20th century, POPs were virtually nonexistent in our environment. Following World War II, the production and distribution of POPs expanded dramatically. Today nearly 900 active ingredients are found in our food, water, homes, schools, and workplaces.[7] These are part of a larger chemical soup of over 60,000 commercially produced synthetic chemicals with about 1,000 new synthetic chemicals being released each year. Each American eats an average of 14 pounds of food additives a year.[8] Some chemicals are more toxic than others, but the cumulative effects make a strong case for banning the use of most additives and all POPs, not just a few of the worst offenders.

POPs accumulate over the course of a lifetime in the bodies of future mothers and fathers. More than 50 percent of the women attending a fertility program in one study had detectable concentrations of environmental toxins in their blood and in the fluids found in their ovaries.[9]

Men too are negatively affected by POPs in terms of sexual abilities and potency.[10] Men in the Midwest with elevated exposure to the commonly used pesticides alachlor, diazinon, and atrazine are significantly more likely to have reduced sperm quality.[11] The United States and Western Europe have seen a dramatic increase in sperm deformities, reducing the ability of sperm to impregnate.[12] European studies done in the early 1990s show a spiraling decline in sperm count.[13] A Scottish study noted, "[There has been] a decline in sperm concentration and the total number of sperm and of motile sperm in the ejaculate in association with a later year of birth, such that men born in the 1970s are producing some 24 percent fewer motile sperm in their ejaculate than are men born in the 1950s."[14] Men's sperm count in Europe and the United States has dropped dramatically since 1938.[15] There is hope, however. A Danish study comparing the sperm counts and diets of a group of airline workers to a group of organic farmers found that the organic farmers, whose diet was at least 25 percent organic, had 43 percent higher sperm counts.[16]

The placental connection to the mother exposes her fetus to environmental pollutants. These POPs disrupt the activities of estrogen, androgen, and thyroid hormones during critical periods of fetal development. The damage from this disruption can show up later in life in the form of altered social skills, decreased intelligence, and reproductive difficulties.[17] Examinations of boys age 16 and older who had been exposed in the womb to polychlorinated biphenyls (PCBs) and dibenzofurans were compared with unexposed counterparts. The results revealed a significant effect on the sperm quality of the boys exposed to the chemicals, with increases in the percentage of abnormally formed sperm, decreases in sperm motility, and decreases in sperm strength.[18] It is not advisable for a pregnant or nursing woman to do the Weekend Cleanse. It is possible that toxins released from fat cells and the liver can cross the placental barrier or be passed to the baby through the mother's milk. Pregnant women should maintain good communication with their midwife or doctor to ensure proper nutrition (including prenatal vitamins or other supplements as needed), hydration, rest, and the satisfaction of any special needs.

The ideal food for an infant is breast milk. Unfortunately, most infants receive huge quantities of pollutants that the mother has been accumulating all of her life.[19] Breast milk is high in fat and in the chemicals that are attracted to and concentrated in fat.[20] Levels of pesticides may be six to seven times higher in breast milk than in the mother's blood.[21] As much as 20 percent of a mother's lifelong burden of pesticides is fed to her infant during the first three months of breast-feeding.[22] In spite of the contaminants, breast-feeding is wonderful for both babies and mothers. Mother's milk is a primary source of antibodies and friendly bacteria. The mother-child bonding that grows from nursing lasts a lifetime. The nutrients in a mother's milk are essential for her baby and cannot be replicated in a factory. Formula should only be substituted as a last resort when breast-feeding is not possible. Lower levels of some environmental toxins, such as DDT and DDE, have been found in the milk of vegetarian mothers, but stable PCB levels indicate that contaminant sources other than food (possibly air pollution) are involved.[23] We need to take action to keep our bodies clean and work to outlaw the use of toxic environmental pollutants. In countries that have banned or greatly reduced POPs, there is a measurable decline in the levels of these chemicals in mothers' milk.[24]

Infants, whose digestive tracts are not completely formed, have a high probability of food hypersensitivity if they have been fed food other than their mother's milk.[25] The foods typically fed to these infants are products made from cow's milk, wheat, eggs, and soy. These are among the most common food allergens.[26]

Children are especially vulnerable to chemical pollutants. Relative to their body weight, children eat more food, and thus more chemicals, than adults. Estimates are that 50 percent of our lifetime exposure to pesticides occurs before the age of six.[27] Children's bodies are composed of developing tissues that are more sensitive than an adult's to the effects of environmental toxins. Children are not good candidates for the fasting parts of a cleanse. Instead they should be fed adequate amounts of organic plant-based foods.

Many toxins are concentrated and stored in our fatty tissues and the fatty substances in our cell walls. These toxins are fat-soluble, which means they only dissolve in fatty or oily solutions. These toxins may remain lodged in our cells for a lifetime, or they may be released during periods of stress or as a result of exercise and fasting.[28]

A key to keeping POPs out of our bodies is to remove them from our surroundings. Most of these chemicals, an estimated 89–99 percent, gain access to our bodies through food.[29] The foods highest on the food chain (meat, poultry, fish, and dairy products) are the foods with the highest levels of contamination. The reason is simple: the fatty tissues of these animal foods attract and concentrate chemicals. Toxins accumulate as they move up the food chain, resulting in a concentration of chemical threats.

The risk from nonorganically grown plant foods can be lowered. The contamination of plants is often a surface phenomenon resulting from spraying pesticides on the plant or from particles of herbicides carried to the surface of the plant by air or water. Thoroughly washing and peeling plant foods can remove most surface contaminants. Unfortunately many poisons used on agricultural crops are systemic, as they work by entering into the cells of the plant. As there is no special labeling required, there is no easy way to tell if the foods we purchase in the grocery store have been treated with systemic poisons.

The clean-burning carbohydrates found in plants most effectively enhance the body's detoxifying processes.[30] Meat, fish, poultry, and oil offer no carbohydrates. Cheese does have miniscule amounts of carbohydrates, but its fats carry toxins, making it basically useless in terms of cleansing the body. Under-eating the right foods and overeating the wrong foods, and even eating too much of the "right" foods, almost invariably leads to a reduced capacity to deactivate toxic pollutants.

There are two strategies we can take to manage the toxin onslaught. One: Steer clear of environmental contaminants and avoid eating the dangerous chemicals found in and on food. Two: Change our internal chemistry to eliminate toxins already present in the body.

The most effective long-term change we can make is to eat organic produce that is untouched by herbicides, pesticides, fungicides, and petroleum-based fertilizers. Toxins concentrate in the tissues of animals, so avoiding fish and other animal foods will reduce our exposure to those chemical concentrations. Some toxins travel on cholesterol particles.[31] Fortunately there is no cholesterol in the plant kingdom. Thus a low-fat vegetarian diet can reduce the amount of cholesterol in the blood and minimize the toxins that are transported by it. While our strongest defense is to avoid these pollutants in the first place, to stay healthy we must also take effective actions to rid our bodies of the poisonous substances that have already accumulated. Organic plant-based food is a critical component of the Weekend Cleanse.

Nutrition Basics

The human body has a vast capacity for health, which can bring us joy, or illness, which can cause suffering. Our health is limited by forces that are often hard to control—genetics, geography, family dynamics, finances, and a host of others. Despite these potential obstacles, we each have an opportunity and an obligation to strive toward optimal health. When our body is clean and operating at its best, it is easier for us to move forward with our dreams.

Human beings love to eat. During our lifetime each of us will consume an estimated two to three tons of food. The food we take in gives us the energy we need to carry on our daily activities. It also provides the nutrients we require to grow, repair tissues, and nourish our brain and all the systems of our body. Thus eating and the process of digestion hold a central place in the human experience.

People can shovel nearly anything into their mouth and their digestive tract will make every effort to deal with it. But that isn't the way to better health. What we eat has a major influence on our well-being. Animals in the wild consume just the right amount of food to maintain their optimal health. Even when an abundance of their natural food is available they do not get too fat. They do not require great feats of willpower to stop eating when they've consumed their fill. Their bodies, like ours, have evolved to achieve and maintain good digestive health when fed the appropriate diet.

Our bodies have the ability to balance caloric intake with caloric expenditure. But this balancing act can only work properly when the food going into our mouths is the food our bodies are adapted to process. In order to maximize our health we must eat foods consistent with our digestive evolution. This means whole foods—fresh fruits, vegetables, whole grains, beans, nuts, and seeds. Redesigning our menu in terms of the types of food we consume is more important than limiting portion size if we want to maintain this natural balance.[32]

Some foods are critical to our health and pass easily and quickly through our system to help it function optimally. Plant foods are the ones to go for. Not only are whole plant foods rich in vitamins and minerals, they contain compounds that renew our bodies and protect us from cancer and other diseases. Fruits, vegetables, beans, and whole grains are also sources of fiber, which is vital to healthy digestion. Our optimal diet comprises the foods our bodies have evolved to process. These foods sustained our ancestors and were rich in both fiber and nutrients—mainly fruits, vegetables, whole grains, beans, and seeds.[33]

Humans process a variety of feedback mechanisms that signal when we have eaten enough food. One of the primary mechanisms to keep our digestion and weight in balance is the feeling of satiation—the sensation we feel as stretch receptor nerves embedded in the gastrointestinal tissues tell us how much the gut has expanded. Not enough stretch and we still feel hungry. Too much stretch and pain sets in. Another factor in this balancing act are nutrient receptors. Recent studies indicate that the human body has receptors for the three macronutrients—carbohydrates, fats, and protein.[34]

So where does caloric density fit in? Fiber and water are essentially calorie free. Carbohydrates and proteins are strikingly similar in caloric density—both contain about 1,800 calories per pound. Fat is the heavyweight in the macronutrient trio; it carries 4,000 calories per pound. In order to moderate our hunger drive, the body determines how much we have eaten based on our stomach's stretch sensation and the caloric density of the food consumed, and signals a sense of hunger or fullness.[35] Additionally, the body monitors fat stores. When fat stores have reached adequate levels, the brain's appetite regulating centers are alerted and the hunger drive is decreased.[36]

Our ancestral diet was probably 10–20 percent fat. Today the standard American diet is 20–40 percent fat. When compared to the standard American diet of 1980, Americans today eat 13 pounds more oil per year. While our diets were increasing in fat, why didn't our bodies signal the sensation of hunger to stop? How did Americans become so overweight? Lack of fiber is the culprit.[37]

Fiber and Carbohydrates

Carbohydrates provide us with two critical ingredients for healthy digestion—fuel and fiber. Examples of popular carbohydrate foods include pancakes, breads, spaghetti, cakes, cookies, and rice. All carbohydrates are composed of carbon, hydrogen, and oxygen. A carbohydrate molecule typically has two atoms of hydrogen for every atom of carbon.

The smallest carbohydrates are simple sugars shaped into tiny molecular rings, usually composed of five or six atoms of carbon and one atom of oxygen. These sugar rings are called monosaccharides. The most common monosaccharide is glucose. Glucose is the primary cellular fuel of humans and most other organisms. We need glucose and we need carbohydrates. We normally have glucose stored as glycogen in our liver and muscles. Our bodies draw on this stored energy as needed. When the reserves get low we feel hungry.

Inside our cells a chemical reaction combines the monosaccharides like small building blocks, forming them into larger carbohydrate molecules. In plants, any two monosaccharides can combine to form a disaccharide. Table sugar, also known as disaccharide sucrose, is synthesized from the monosaccharides fructose and glucose. When three or more monosaccharides are joined, they form large carbohydrate molecules called polysaccharides. Non-starch polysaccharides include mucilage, pectin, and gums—water-soluble hemicelluloses that can form stable gels.

Polysaccharides form the basis of plant starch and the plant fiber called cellulose. Both starch and cellulose are long chains of thousands of glucose molecules. The critical difference between starch and cellulose is in how the glucose molecules are bound.

When we eat and digest the starch polysaccharide, water, with the help of a specific enzyme in our digestive system, splits the long molecules into smaller molecules. This chemical reaction is called hydrolysis. Hydrolysis makes the food molecules easier to absorb. This is an important part of digestion. Hydrolysis does not break down the polysaccharide cellulose because humans don't have the necessary enzyme.

Cellulose, the most abundant molecule produced by living systems, is one type of dietary fiber. Cellulose fiber gives plant cells structural support. It is a major component of brown rice, whole wheat, carrots, leafy green vegetables, and most other plant material in our diet.

The current American diet has only a fraction of the fiber found in our ancestral diet. Although dieticians generally recommend getting 20–30 grams of fiber daily, most Americans get about 10–18 grams a day.[38] Fiber consumption before the last century had been between 40 and 70 grams a day. The World Health Organization recommends that most adults eat 27–40 grams of fiber each day. This comes to 15–22 grams of fiber for each 1,000 kcal. Kcal is the an abbreviation for kilogram calorie; a kilocalorie is the quantity of energy needed to raise the temperature

Plant Fiber

Cellulose fibrils can be found in the cell walls of plant cells. The fibrils are made of bundled tubes of microfibrils.

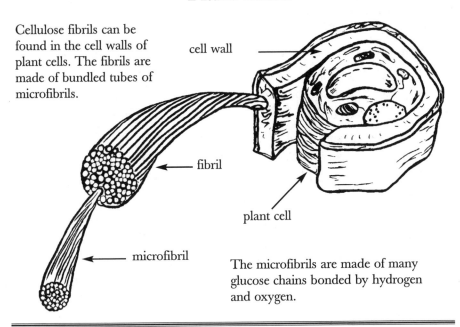

cell wall

fibril

plant cell

microfibril

The microfibrils are made of many glucose chains bonded by hydrogen and oxygen.

of a kilogram of water from 14.5°C to 15.5°C. Thus Americans consuming 2,000–2,800 kcal per day need to eat 30–62 grams of fiber each day.[39] Those who are already eating a vegetarian diet are probably getting 30–40 grams of fiber per day. If vegetarians adhere to a dairy-free and egg-free vegan diet, the daily average is likely in the range of 40–50 grams of fiber.[40]

Fiber does not register on the nutrient receptors that monitor the caloric density of protein, carbohydrates, and fat, but fiber is a major presence in the digestive system. By stimulating the stretch receptor sites in the gastrointestinal tract, fiber plays a role in how the body determines when enough has been consumed. Foods with low fiber and high fat disrupt the system and result in an increase in calories per volume of food ingested. With less plant fiber there is less bulk relative to the number of calories consumed. Overeating is the immediate result. Continued overeating not only impairs digestion and bowel function, it also increases the risk of heart disease, stroke, diabetes, and obesity.[41]

There are two forms of fiber: soluble fiber and insoluble fiber. Soluble fiber is most abundant in beans, oats, and fruit. Softer stools result from the consumption of soluble fiber because it absorbs up to 15 times its weight in water while moving through the digestive tract. Soluble fibers—the non-starch polysaccharides (water-soluble hemicelluloses) such as mucilage, pectin, and gums—are partially broken down by our intestinal bacteria. These characteristics of soluble fiber are a gift to our digestive system, as this type of fiber helps sweep our intestines clean.

Insoluble fiber is composed of the structural elements of plants: cellulose and lignin. These fibers attract and soak up water and are unlikely to dissolve.[42] Insoluble fiber is not broken down into its component glucose molecules because our digestive enzymes cannot break the linkage between the glucose molecules. Insoluble fiber passes into the feces in its original form. Without enough insoluble fiber in the diet the feces become hardened, making it more difficult for them to move through the nearly 30 feet of intestines. Ominously, small pockets and bulges called diverticula are created by the intense muscular contractions required to move the feces. The final expelling of the low-fiber stool requires a strong squeeze that frequently causes hemorrhoids.[43]

Stool receives its bulk from the insoluble fiber found in vegetables, legumes (peas, beans, and lentils), and whole grains. Plants are virtually our sole source of this critical dietary fiber. The only animal products with fiber are the membranes of some shellfish. As for red meat, eggs, cheese, and chicken, there is no fiber at all. Refined flour and refined grains have had most of their precious fiber removed.[44] People who adopt a vegetarian diet that includes whole grains automatically increase their intake of insoluble fiber.

The softening and bulking of stools produced by these two types of fiber help prevent a host of ailments including constipation, some types of diarrhea, and some of the symptoms of irritable bowel syndrome (IBS). The passage of fiber actually reduces pressure on the intestinal walls, lessening the risk of diverticular disease and hemorrhoids. Cholesterol may be lowered due to the increased amount of bile acids excreted into the stool. The liver creates bile acids, in part by removing cholesterol from the bloodstream. Diabetes may be better controlled with the consumption of fiber because fiber slows the release of sugar into the bloodstream. Although current research has not yet determined whether the benefit for those with diabetes is directly from the fiber itself or because a high-fiber diet is usually low in fat and high in nutrients that may help control blood sugar, the course of action is clear: eat high-fiber foods.

When upping the fiber content of the diet, it is advisable to increase the amounts gradually. In certain circumstances it is possible to have too much fiber in the diet. Too much too quickly can cause gas and bloating. Going more slowly will give the intestinal flora an opportunity to adjust.

Children, with their small stomachs and appetites, may need more concentrated food energy than a heavily fibrous diet might provide. Elderly people, who may have limited appetites, also need concentrated calories. Cooking fibrous foods can be beneficial for the very young and the elderly, because heat breaks down fiber, making it softer and less filling.[45]

Although fiber had been long recognized as a valued part of the diet, fiber achieved new status in America in the 1800s when the Christian evangelist Sylvester Graham added fiber to his enthusiasms. The namesake product he created—graham crackers—remains popular to this day.

In 1875 new milling techniques allowed the removal of bran and wheat germ from flour. This white flour was a big hit with consumers who enjoyed the taste and texture of the new food. Manufacturers and grocery store owners liked the longer shelf life of the processed grains and the concurrent increase in profitability. Unfortunately the eliminated bran and wheat germ contained most of the fiber and substantial amounts of iron, zinc, magnesium, vitamin E, and the B vitamins. In a short time some of the negative health results of the new milling process became obvious, and iron and a portion of the B vitamins were added back into the flour. This attempt to replace the grain's natural balance of nutrients resulted in an "enriched" flour, a product nutritionally inferior to whole grain flour.[46]

Sister Ellen White, an influential Seventh-day Adventist who in 1866 established the Battle Creek Sanitarium in Battle Creek, Michigan, took up the fiber banner. A commercial spin-off from the deepening understanding of the role of fiber later came out of the Battle Creek Sanitarium when two employees, W. K. Kellogg and Dr. John Harvey Kellogg, who championed plant-based diets, developed Kellogg breakfast cereals. Kellogg's Corn Flakes appeared in the market in 1906. Kellogg's All Bran came out in 1916 under the name Krumbled Bran, with the explicit label, "Relieves Constipation."[47] The descendants of those early breakfast cereals can still be found on grocery store shelves.[48]

The 20th century saw a widespread use of denatured flours and grains. Coming out of the Great Depression of the 1930s, American prosperity favored the increased consumption of fats and meats. A meal came to be considered "incomplete" if there was no meat served. Bowel disorders and related diseases increased.[49]

Proteins

Proteins are among the most important components of our food. Our cells use protein as raw material to regenerate and build new tissues. When cells have exhausted their supplies of carbohydrates and lipids they harvest proteins for necessary energy. The need for protein is a well-advertised rallying cry for the multitrillion-dollar meat industry. "I need more protein so I need more meat" is the adage of many who are constipated, overweight, dealing with clogged arteries, and reeling from one sickness to the next.

The function of a protein depends on its type, and each type has a unique shape. The shape of protein is formed in a marvelous and not yet fully understood chemical dance. Protein consists of large macromolecules made up of thousands of atoms. Twenty different amino acids form the building blocks of protein. Two or more amino acids can be joined by peptide bonds like a molecular jigsaw puzzle. The molecule formed when two amino acids are joined by peptide bonds is called a dipeptide. When three or more amino acids are connected by peptide bonds the new molecule is a polypeptide chain. Proteins are long polypeptide chains averaging 200 amino acids per chain. Proteins are differentiated from one another by the order of the various kinds of amino acids in the polypeptide chain.

The vast majority of enzymes are proteins that act as catalysts to increase the rate of activity and change inside a cell. They are essential to the digestion of food and the regulation of a cell's metabolism. Enzymes make efficient use of energy to create change inside a cell. The minimum energy needed to generate a particular reaction inside a cell is called the activation energy. An enzyme's particular value comes from its shape. The place where the shape of an enzyme and a substrate molecule fit together is called the active site. The substrate is the molecule acted upon. Enzymes do not usually finish their task without help from a cofactor, such as a metal ion or an organic molecule called a coenzyme. Both the structure and function of a cell is dependent on the enzymes it produces.

The secretion of digestive enzymes is reduced when the body is in a horizontal position. This is one of the problems with eating late at night. Buddha advised his students, "Not eating a meal at night, I am aware of good health and of being without illness and [having] buoyancy and strength and living in comfort. Come, you too, do not eat at night."[50] The exact role of enzymes may not have been known during the time of the Buddha, but the benefits of not sleeping on a full stomach were.

Fats, Oils, and Lipids

Fat is a greasy, semisolid material found in both animals and plants. Excess fat in the diet slows digestion, causing heartburn, bloating, and constipation. Worse yet, excess fat raises our risk for a number of debilitating and even life-threatening health conditions such as heart disease, diabetes, and gallbladder diseases. The symptoms of irritable bowel syndrome, pancreatitis, and Crohn's disease are all magnified by excess dietary fat. The exact mechanism is unclear, but research gathered by the American Institute for Cancer Research implicates dietary fat in the promotion of colon cancer, gallbladder cancer, and other cancers.[51]

Our body fat is a collection of large lipid droplets stored in fat cells. Lipids are important components of food that do not dissolve in water. Lipids are found in vegetable oil, butter, and margarine, and even in household products like furniture wax. Much of the value of lipids is in their insolubility. Lipids are used as a protective barrier between the cell and the watery interior environment filled with all those water-soluble molecules. Lipids also store energy. When needed for fuel, these drops of lipids are broken down to provide energy.

Most fat is made of molecules called triglycerides. Triglycerides are three fatty acid molecules held together by a three-carbon alcohol called glycerol. Fatty acids are long chains of carbon atoms with clusters of atoms called carboxyl groups at the ends of the chains. Each of the carbon atoms in the chain has the possibility of bonding with two hydrogen atoms. If the maximum number of hydrogen atoms is attached to the carbon atoms, the fatty acid molecule is called saturated. Saturated fats occur naturally or are artificially produced by hydrogenation of fats. Those fats with fewer hydrogen atoms attached are called unsaturated. Some fatty acids have more than two double bonds and are said to be polyunsaturated. Saturated fatty acids are solid at room temperature and can be found in lard and butter. Triglycerides, made of unsaturated fatty acids, are liquid at room temperature and are called oils. Although there are exceptions to the rule, animal products are likely to have saturated fats, while plant foods contain unsaturated oils. Exceptions include palm oil and coconut oil, which come from plants yet are highly saturated. Saturated fats are harder to digest and are usually stored as fat.[52] To protect your health, limit your intake of fats in general and hydrogenated and saturated fats in particular.

Fluids

Drinking ample amounts of fluids is important for healthy digestion. Water is the best fluid, although most beverages, such as herbal tea and juice, are more than 90 percent water. The liquids that do not help are beer, wine, and hard liquor. For many years it was thought that caffeinated drinks acted as diuretics and actually increased fluid loss by increasing urine volume. A review of current research reported in the *International Journal of Sport Nutrition Exercise and Metabolism* suggests that drinking caffeinated drinks does not cause detrimental fluid loss or any electrolyte imbalance.[53]

Fluids help by lubricating food as it passes along its digestive journey. Water-softened stools help prevent constipation. Fluids also increase nutrient absorption by dissolving minerals and fat-soluble vitamins such as vitamins A, D, E, and K.

If you are uncertain if you are drinking enough liquids for good digestion, you can check the color and odor of your urine. This can be done by first washing the urinary opening and collecting a "clean-catch" (midstream) urine sample. Clear the urethra of contaminants by first passing a little urine into the toilet bowl. Then catch two or three finger widths of urine in a clean glass. Take a look and have a whiff.

A pale yellow color going out indicates enough liquid is going in. Dark yellow urine that smells of ammonia indicates a need to increase fluid intake. Bacterial infections of the kidneys or bladder will give urine a foul smell. Musty smelling urine indicates liver disease and, in rare cases, it

Urine Odor	Possible Cause
ammonia	dehydration
foul	kidney or bladder infection
musty	liver disease, phenylketonuria
sweet	diabetes
maple syrup	maple sugar urine disease
other	medications, asparagus, Vitamin B_{12}

may indicate phenylketonuria, an inherited metabolic disorder.[54] If odd smelling urine is accompanied by other symptoms, get the opinion of a health care professional. If your urine is pink or bloody, medical help is required. (In some people, beets can cause urine to turn red or fuchsia.)

If urine is passed fewer than four times a day, more fluids are called for. If you have trouble urinating or if you are going so often that you are dehydrated, a health care professional should be consulted.

Causes of Blood in the Urine (hematuria)

bladder diseases:
   bladder cancer
   bladder papilloma
cervical cancer
cystitis
diabetic nephropathy
immune thrombocytopenic
   purpura
internal injury
kidney diseases:
   acute kidney failure
   autosomal dominant
     polycystic kidney disease
   cystic kidney disease
   glomerular disease
   kidney cancer

kidney stones
nephritis
polycystic kidney disease
pyelonephritis
malaria
porphyria
prostate cancer
prostate enlargement
prostatitis
renal colic
schistosomiasis
thalassemia
thrombocytopenia
urinary stones
urinary tract infections
Wilms' tumor

THE
Digestive Tract

A discussion of proper cleansing and an understanding of the Weekend Cleanse must start with an overview of the workings of the digestive system. The digestive system is wonderfully flexible and can adjust to a wide range of foods and stressful experiences. This ability is hardwired into our bodies by millions of years of evolutionary trial and error. Digestion—taking in food and breaking it down into usable parts— was one of the early vital life functions that evolved in our one-celled ancestors.[1] The association of cells for mutual benefit grew from colonies of bacteria. Those communities that were successful reproduced—tweaking and fine-tuning the process. Eventually these colonies developed specialized functions.

Some of the earliest complex life forms consisted primarily of self-maintaining digestive tubes. Nutrients entered the "head" end of the tube and waste material exited the other end. Between these two ends, cells harvested needed molecules. Life prospered, filling more niches. Special cells evolved that coordinated movement. The collection of food became response driven as neural systems grew to inform the expanding repertoire of possibilities.

The Digestive Tract

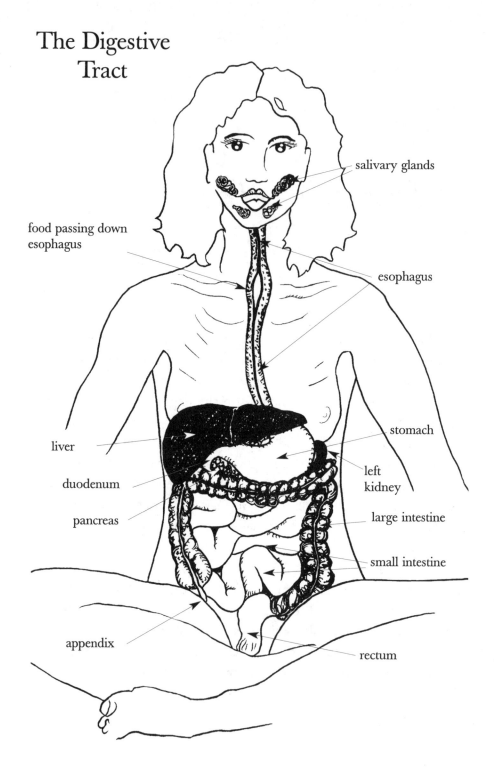

salivary glands

food passing down esophagus

esophagus

liver

stomach

duodenum

left kidney

pancreas

large intestine

small intestine

appendix

rectum

We can only speculate about the digestive health of the preliterate world. Certain changes can be tracked by archaeologists, such as the disease or health of bones and teeth and the remains of meals and harvests found at ancient sites. During the 3.5 million years when our ancestors lived as scavengers, gatherers, and hunters, our communities were small. People lived as nomads and seminomadic groups of perhaps 200–250 people. Then someone, most likely a woman, began gathering and planting seeds.[2] A stabilization of the food supply was possible. Grains, nuts, root crops, and dried foods could be stored for difficult times when food might be hard to come by. The advent of agriculture in human communities brought forth civilization. Agriculture also affected our digestion and nutrition in ways we are still discovering. Dietary paleontologists are in general agreement that our ancestral diet was mainly fruits, vegetables, whole grains, beans, and seeds. These foods have high essential nutrient levels packed into calories laced with fiber.[3]

Although food selection has always been a part of human life, a studied understanding of the deeper relationship between digestion and health seems to have come in fits and starts. Today, imaging techniques such as CAT scans, ultrasound, PET scans, colonoscopy, endoscopy, and capsule endoscopy give us incredible insight into the actual positioning and living action of the intestines.

Digestion

Food enters the mouth and is digested, absorbed, and eliminated—touching a universe of convoluted surfaces. Together these surfaces form a large and primary interface with a vital source of life: the food we eat. This interfacing interior gut has some of the highest concentrations of protective immune cells in the body. During food's journey through the elaborate tube of our intestines, it is exposed to a cocktail of digestive enzymes. Each enzyme speeds up the reactions that break the food into useable molecules.

Digestion is a function of an organ system. Its role is to acquire materials and energy by digesting food into small molecules and then absorbing those molecules. The digestive system is neurologically rich, containing more nerve cells than the spine. Much of digestion is controlled by an autonomous nervous system—the "enteric" nervous system—that can function independently of the brain. There are five processes that are involved with digestion: eating, breaking down food into simpler chemical compounds, absorption, assimilation, and elimination of waste. Our food choices play a significant role in the quality of our digestion. Although chewing and saliva begin the process, the bulk of our food is broken down in the stomach and small intestine. Absorption is when molecules pass into our bloodstream. Assimilation is when those molecules enter our cells. Elimination of waste is the job of the colon, lymph, lungs, kidneys, and skin.

The nose also contributes to healthy digestion. We are favored with an open nose interior lined with receptors that interpret the oils and other oxidizing factors exuded by our food.[4] The response of receptors to the aromas indicates the appropriateness of the food for us. We are attracted to some odors and repelled by others. The subtleness of the aroma receptors protecting our digestive system is astounding. The Nobel Prize in medicine, announced in October 2004, went to two scientists who studied how humans are able to recognize and recall 10,000 distinct scents.[5] The potential of the nose for discerning the safety of foods may be greater than that—there are accounts of two physicians during the time of Buddha who together could identify 108,000 scents.[6]

Few organs are more exquisitely adapted to bring pleasure to humans than the tongue. The tongue has pressure regulators similar to the pressure receptors in our skin. The tongue is also loaded with chemical receptors called taste buds that, under magnification, look like the buds of delicate flowers. Additional taste buds are found on the surface of the mouth and throat. The range of information revealed by our nose and taste buds—sweet, sour, salty, pungent, bitter, tart, tangy—exceeds even the input from our skin. We can do our tongues a favor and refresh our taste buds by cleaning the residue from the tongue's surface with a tongue scraper.

The Abdominal Region

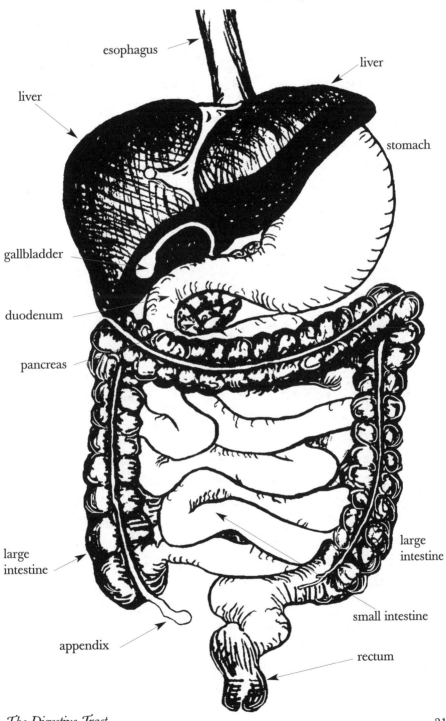

esophagus

liver

liver

stomach

gallbladder

duodenum

pancreas

large
intestine

large
intestine

small intestine

appendix

rectum

The Digestive Tract

The muscular tongue pushes and directs the food to the teeth. The teeth tear and crush the food, increasing the food's surface area and mixing it with saliva. For maximum digestion, food should be chewed thoroughly. Some macrobiotic sources recommend chewing each mouthful of food at least 50 times for a healthy individual and 150 times for someone with cancer.[7] That may be a difficult regimen to maintain, but even occasional counting of chews can be beneficial. Overstuffing the mouth and swallowing food before it is sufficiently broken down by teeth and saliva is a common source of mild indigestion (dyspepsia) and flatulence.[8]

When teeth are missing, or if teeth and gums are painful, chewing food can be difficult, making this early step in digestion inadequate. Regular dental care including flossing and brushing are critical to maintaining healthy gums and strong teeth free of cavities and pain.

Three pairs of salivary glands send streams of saliva through ducts and into the mouth. Saliva is rich in the enzyme called salivary amylase. Salivary amylase begins the digestion of starches. To get a sense of this, thoroughly chew a bite of bread, without swallowing, and taste the sweetness as the carbohydrates are broken down into sugars. There was an interesting examination of the effects of meditation on the quality of saliva. Twelve dental students had the bacteria levels and consistency of their saliva tested before and after 20 minutes of meditation. The post-meditation saliva had changed from opaque to translucent with a reduction in the levels of bacteria.[9]

Swallowing moves the chewed food down the esophagus, through a muscular door called the lower esophageal sphincter, and into the stomach. There are two troubling symptoms that can appear while swallowing that require the attention of a health care professional. One symptom is when a swallow of food seems to lodge in the chest and won't go down. This distressful sensation often occurs with the first bite of a meal and may last several minutes. Another symptom, also likely to appear at the beginning of a meal, is the feeling of a muscle spasm in the center of the stomach accompanied by a feeling of nausea. These symptoms, which may appear only occasionally, can be caused by a difficulty in swallowing (dysphagia). Dysphagia can be caused by a growth in the esophagus, peptic disorders, stress, or irregular esophageal spasms called esophageal dysmotility. Diagnosis by a professional is called for before choosing a course of action. For some, dietary modification is all that is needed; in other cases medication or even surgery may be necessary.[10]

Heartburn and Acid Reflux Disease

The continual bathing of the esophagus with stomach acid can cause chronic heartburn known as gastroesophageal reflux disease (GERD). This can predispose people to esophageal cancer. Heartburn is often first felt as a burning sensation behind the breastbone that radiates up toward the neck. A sour or bitter taste may enter the mouth accompanied by a taste of the offending food. In the United States, heartburn has reached epidemic proportions. The American College of Gastroenterology estimates that more than 60 million Americans experience heartburn at least once a month, and some studies have suggested that more than 15 million Americans experience heartburn symptoms daily.[11] The discomfort from heartburn can interfere with sleep.

Overweight people are more likely to suffer from bloating, constipation, and gastroesophageal reflux disease than thin people. Excess weight increases pressure within and on the abdomen, forcing stomach acid up into the esophagus (acid reflux) causing heartburn and inflaming the delicate tissues lining the esophagus. Noting which foods cause heartburn and avoiding them will reduce symptoms, as will quitting smoking and not drinking alcohol. Chronic acid reflux disease can lead to a number of worsening conditions such as Barrett's esophagus, erosive esophagitis, esophageal strictures, and esophageal cancer.

The United States has a $13 billion-a-year antacid industry. Some of these acid-suppressing drugs have provided relief for millions of discomforted people. However a study published in the *Journal of the American Medical Association* in October 2004 casts doubt on the safety record of these drugs.[12] The research conducted by Robert J. F. Laheji, PhD, of the

Villus (a single villi of the intestinal lining)

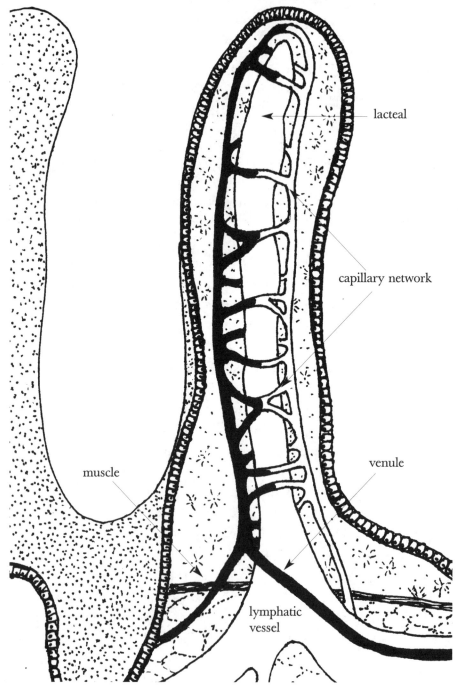

lacteal

capillary network

venule

muscle

lymphatic
vessel

University Medical Center St. Radboud in the Netherlands, involved 364,700 Dutch patients. The results showed that those taking acid-suppressing drugs developed pneumonia four times more often than patients who never took the drugs. To adjust for the fact that those inclined to take acid-suppressing drugs tend to be less healthy, the researchers compared people who used to take the drugs but stopped with people who were still taking them. Those who were still taking acid-suppressants were twice as likely to develop pneumonia. The reason appears to be that stomach acid protects the body from gastrointestinal pathogens, and the acid suppressants reduced the acid levels in the stomach. Just how pneumonia-causing bacteria and viruses move from the stomach into the lungs is not clear. The elderly tend to be the major consumers of acid-suppressing drugs. For them pneumonia can be deadly.[13] Those taking acid-suppressing drugs should be aware of the early warning signs of pneumonia: a fever, usually over 100.5 degrees, accompanied by a cough, especially a productive (wet or phlegm) cough. Additional early signs of pneumonia may include shortness of breath without exertion and a chest pain made worse with deep breathing.

Some protection against cancerous esophageal cells comes from a strange relationship called the "*pylori* paradox."[14] More than half the earth's population harbors the bacteria *Heliobacter pylori* in their stomach. Certain strains of *H. pylori* are particularly implicated in triggering stomach ulcers and cancers. Stomach cancer is the second most common of the deadly cancers. The odd thing is that those same strains of the bacteria produce a protein known as CagA that appears to be protective against esophageal cancer. The troubling implication is that treating *H. pylori* with antibiotics may increase the risk of esophageal cancer.

We owe our ability to periodically eat "good-sized" meals and then get involved in unrelated activities to the storage capacity of our stomachs. The stomach can, under normal circumstances, store two or more liters of partially digested food.

Digestive juices flow from the walls of the stomach and small intestines, pancreas, and gallbladder. Enzymes, bile, and bacteria break down the food. Our food, for all of our kitchen magic, consists mostly of fats, proteins, and the fiber, starches, and sugars known as carbohydrates. Some of these are bound in complex molecules that are snipped by enzymes into smaller, simpler strings of atoms. Deeper in the intestines, bacteria digest and release food nutrients. At some point the size, structure, and content of the snipped nutrient molecules allow them entry into and through the 50–100 trillion cells that constitute the living wonder of our organs, nerves, and consciousness.

The breaking down of food takes place in the digestive system, and the reassembly takes place once cells throughout the body receive the products of digestion. Enzymes break down the starches and complex sugars into simple sugars. Fats are divided by enzymes into fatty acids and glycerol. Enzymes reduce the proteins to their component amino acids. The amino acids, themselves the building blocks of protein, are reassembled into new protein by a series of wonderfully intricate chemical exchanges. The processes create the "physical" platform that is constantly becoming the body. Who can fail to be amazed?

The Western world gained unique insight into the workings of the stomach when a French Canadian named Alexis St. Martin was shot in the abdomen in 1822.[15] Dr. William Beaumont, the U.S. Army doctor who treated St. Martin, was a meticulous observer. St. Martin's wound healed around an open hole that enabled Beaumont, for the next eight years, to look inside the stomach and observe the walls of the stomach contracting violently to mix the food and gastric juices containing hydrochloric acid (HCl) and pepsin. Beaumont was the first to observe that the gastric juices and the protective mucous secretions of the stomach are produced independently of each other. Before that, medical science had few clues about what happened to food after it was swallowed.

Food in the stomach is processed by hydrochloric acid, which has an intensely acidic pH of 2.0. That is strong enough to kill most bacteria and other organisms that may have been consumed with the food. The acid also stops the activity of the saliva that had been working on the food up to this point.

The activities of the stomach convert the food into a thick, soupy mass called chyme. Chyme releases most of its nutrients after leaving the stomach and entering the small intestine. Although called "small," this portion of the digestive tract, if it were spread flat, would cover a surface the size of a tennis court. The small intestine is a membrane moistened constantly by mucus-secreting goblet cells. The mucus performs three important functions. It protects the intestinal wall from digestive enzymes. Mucus provides a safe haven for the friendly bacteria that are so vital to our health. Additionally, the secreted mucous lubricates the food, chyme, and feces on the voyage. The small intestine is guarded by immune system cells to protect us from toxins that have passed through our mouths.

The surface of the small intestine is marked by 4–5 million small, finger-like projections called villi. These villi absorb the products of digestion (see the villus illustration on page 34). Each individual villus contains blood vessels surrounding a connection to the lymph system, a lymphatic capillary called a lacteal. Nutrients diffuse through the exterior cells of the villi and pass through the capillary walls and the lacteal to enter the circulatory system and the lymphatic system.

There are three main sections of the small intestine: the duodenum, jejunum, and the ileum. The base of the stomach is gated by a sphincter muscle that relaxes and contracts, squirting small amounts of chyme into the first 12–18 inches of the small intestine, the active, mucus-layered tube called the duodenum. Here is where pancreatic juice and enzymes come in contact with the chyme. Numerous nutrients are released from the chyme and passed into the blood, including vitamins B_1, B_2, B_6, and C; the minerals calcium, magnesium, iron, zinc, copper, and manganese; glucose; galactose; fructose; fats; and the fat-soluble vitamins A, D, and E.

The duodenum is a location where ulcers and other types of digestive stress can manifest. Sudden stress causes the adrenal glands to secrete hormones that reduce the supply of blood to the digestive tract and increase the blood supply to the muscles.[16] Long-term, low-level stress can deplete the adrenal glands, wreck our digestion, and leave us with that "wiped out" feeling. Fortunately, stress-related problems usually can be reversed.

In a normally healthy person, a thick layer of mucus protects the walls of the stomach and duodenum. If gastric acid gets through the mucus, the pepsin in the gastric juices begins to actually digest the duodenum, creating an ulcer.

Smooth muscle moves material through the digestive tract. Smooth muscle fibers are composed of layers of spindle-shaped cells in which the thick middle portion of one cell is opposite the ends of adjacent cells.

The duodenum is followed by 8–10 feet of thick-walled intestine known as the jejunum. Most of the breakdown of foods happens before the beginning of the jejunum. After this, the primary activity of the intestines is absorption. The tissue of the jejunum is rippled with folds rich in blood vessels that are harvesting proteins, amino acids, sucrose, maltose, lactose, and the water-soluble vitamins thiamine, pyridoxine, riboflavin, and folic acid from the river of chyme.

From the jejunum the chyme passes, through an indistinct junction, into the longest portion of the small intestine, the ileum. The ileum is a narrow, thinner-walled tube with fewer folds and blood vessels than the jejunum, and thus fewer interfaces with the chyme. The ileum passes cholesterol, vitamin B_{12}, and bile salts into the bloodstream.

The processing of food and the elimination of wastes and poisons involve every system of the body. Three organs of critical importance to the digestive tract are the liver, gallbladder, and pancreas.

Liver

The liver is a four pound, two-lobed, solid organ that is absolutely essential in breaking down food molecules, reconstituting nutrients, processing vitamins and minerals, and neutralizing poisons. The liver is as critical to detoxification as lungs are to breathing.

You can locate your liver if you put your left hand over the lowest ribs on your front right side. Beneath your hand, concentrated in your liver, is 20 percent of your blood. Half your body's macrophages, critical agents of your immune system, are located here. Many problems can beset the liver, yet it maintains an astounding ability to regenerate itself—even if only 20 percent of the liver survives some calamity.

The Liver

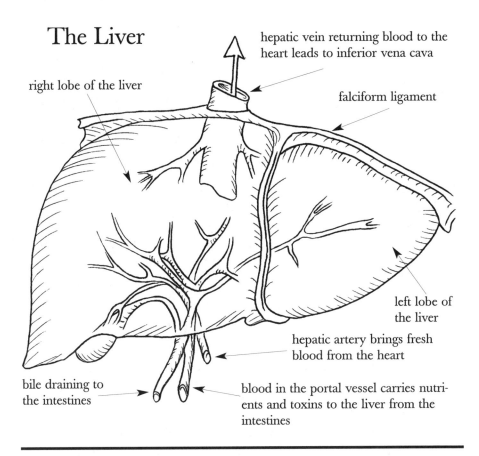

hepatic vein returning blood to the
heart leads to inferior vena cava

right lobe of the liver

falciform ligament

left lobe of
the liver

hepatic artery brings fresh
blood from the heart

bile draining to
the intestines

blood in the portal vessel carries nutrients and toxins to the liver from the
intestines

What is happening in the liver? Both toxins and nutrients absorbed in
the gastrointestinal tract are funneled through the portal vessel and into
the liver. The cells of the liver produce 13,000 powerful enzymes. Toxic
chemicals are carried to the liver where they are met by enzymes catalyz-
ing hundreds of biochemical reactions that neutralize poisons.

Getting rid of fat-soluble poisons is a two-phase job that the enzymes
pull off in a fraction of a second. It works like this: In phase 1 an enzyme
delivers an oxygen molecule to the toxic particle. The oxygen molecule
allows a second enzyme, the phase 2 enzyme, to attach the toxic particle
to a larger carrier molecule that takes the poisons off to the stool, urine,
and bile.

Unfortunately there are cancer-producing toxins that can be activated by the phase 1 enzyme. The point in this exchange that is most danger-ous is right after the phase 1 enzyme has attached the oxygen atom to the toxic molecule. Oxygen is highly reactive. If a phase 2 enzyme does not snatch up the carcinogen and stick it to a carrier molecule, the toxin can damage a person's DNA—triggering the cascading disaster of cancer.

Fortunately it is here that we can take action to make a difference. The critical factor is having lots of phase 2 enzymes present to render the carcinogens and other poisons harmless. The secret is that certain vegetables supply naturally occurring compounds that stimulate the liver to make more phase 2 enzymes. Research by Paul Talalay, MD, of Johns Hopkins University School of Medicine shows that cruciferous plants (cabbage, broccoli, cauliflower, Brussels sprouts, kale, and others) are rich in chemicals that increase the production of phase 2 enzymes.[17] The most effective are Brussels sprouts and green cabbage. Other valuable sources of phase 2 enzyme stimulants are soybeans and soy products including tofu, tempeh, and soymilk.

When the phase 2 enzyme attaches the toxin to a carrier molecule, that molecule is most often glutathione. The next line of defense we have con-trol over is to supply the liver with lots of glutathione. The best sources of glutathione are raw vegetables and raw fruits. Foods richest in glu-tathione are asparagus, avocados, broccoli, garlic, okra, and spinach.[18] Eat them in abundance. Broccoli's dual roles in stimulating phase 2 enzymes and supplying glutathione has won it an honored place in can-

---

SOURCES OF PHASE 2 ENZYME STIMULANTS

broccoli	seitan
Brussels sprouts	soybeans
cauliflower	soymilk
green cabbage	tempeh
kale	tofu

Simple Cleanse

cer prevention. The powerful antioxidant milk thistle can prevent glutathione depletion. The active compound in milk thistle is silymarin, a natural liver detoxifier that protects the liver from poisons like alcohol and carbon tetrachloride.[19] Milk thistle is available as a supplement in most health food stores.

The liver, among its other functions, produces a green fluid called bile that breaks down fats. Bile flows from the liver into the duodenum. Additional bile secreted by the liver is stored in the gallbladder, which is later passed, as needed, through a narrow duct into the duodenum where it is quickly used for digestion. (See the illustration of the liver on page 39 and the pancreas on page 47.)

Where does the liver get bile? After nutrients have entered the bloodstream they arrive at the liver. Some nutrients are stored in the liver, while others are assembled into more complex compounds. Some of these compounds form the liquid bile. Other nutrients and complex compounds are released by the liver and transported throughout the body. They find their way into the nourishing fluids that surround and bathe the cells. From there they enter the cell.

Sadly, 40,000 Americans die from liver disease each year. Sometimes signs of a compromised liver are revealed in the skin: acne, rashes, dark circles under the eyes, liver spots, yellowing of the skin. Other warning signs are revealed in the mouth such as a white coating on the tongue, a bitter taste between meals, and bad breath. The emotions also come into play. Melancholy is derived from the Greek *melas* (black) plus *chole* (bile) or "black bile." Depression and anxiety can accompany liver dysfunction.[20]

One of the most important decisions that can be made to help the liver is to not stress it. Some manufactured chemicals may be comparatively harmless, but others can be highly toxic. Although some chemicals are relatively easy for the liver to process, studies that examine the effects of the random mixtures of chemicals that find their way into our livers from processed food and industrial farming practices are difficult to conduct.[21] To be safe, avoid synthetic chemicals. Fried foods, such as french fries and fried chicken, are typically cooked in overheated hydrogenated fats.

THE LIVER LOVER'S LIST

alfalfa	vitamin K
amaranth	methionine
apples	antioxidants
asparagus	glutathione, essential fatty acids, vitamin K
avocados	glutathione, essential fatty acids
beets	antioxidants
berries	antioxidants
broccoli	glutathione, sulfur compounds
brown rice	arginine, essential fatty acids, selenium
Brussels sprouts	essential fatty acids, sulfur compounds
cabbage	sulfur compounds, vitamin K
carob	arginine
carrots	antioxidants
cauliflower	sulfur compounds
celery	antioxidants
chocolate	arginine
citrus fruits	antioxidants
cold-pressed oils	essential fatty acids
garlic	glutathione, methionine, selenium, sulfur compounds, vitamin K
kale	methionine
leafy greens	essential fatty acids, vitamin K
leeks	sulfur compounds
legumes	methionine
lentils	arginine
melons	antioxidants
molasses	selenium
nuts	essential fatty acids
okra	glutathione
onions	methionine
pears	antioxidants
peas	arginine, antioxidants
sesame seeds	methionine
shallots	sulfur compounds
spinach	antioxidants, glutathione, essential fatty acids, vitamin K
sunflower seeds	methionine
tahini	methionine
tomatoes	vitamin K
walnuts	arginine, essential fatty acids
whole grains	essential fatty acids, selenium

Foods like this place a heavy burden on the liver because they are sources of lipid peroxides (rancid fats) and trans-fatty acids. Lipid peroxides suppress the immune system and damage liver cell membranes. Trans-fatty acids suppress production of the liver-protecting anti-inflammatory prostaglandin, PGE1.[22] (Prostaglandins are a class of chemical messengers derived from fatty acids.) Reduce and avoid greasy foods.

After a good tweaking and purifying of the intestinal tract, the liver ought to be cleansed. The gentle way to do this is to eat liver-friendly foods that benefit liver function. The liver, in addition to glutathione, needs arginine, essential fatty acids, methionine, selenium, sulfur compounds, vitamin K, and antioxidants.[23]

Arginine is an amino acid required by the liver to detoxify ammonia, a common toxin released by protein metabolism. Arginine is found in brown rice, walnuts, beans, peas, lentils, and chocolate (a pleasant surprise!). Among other benefits, arginine has been used to treat male impotence and female sexual dysfunction.[24] Essential fatty acids are required in plentiful amounts for healthy liver function. We find them in legumes, whole grains, cold-pressed oils, avocados, and fresh nuts. Methionine is a sulfur-containing amino acid essential for detoxification.[25] It is thought to keep fat from building up in the liver.[26] Methionine is found in legumes, garlic, onions, sesame seeds and tahini, sunflower seeds, amaranth, kale, and lentils. Natural sulfur compounds are available from broccoli, Brussels sprouts, cabbage, cauliflower, garlic, leeks, onions, and shallots. Selenium is an antioxidant abundant in brown rice, molasses, whole grains, garlic, and onions. Sulfur compounds increase the activity of the liver's phase 2 detoxification enzymes. Vitamin K is found in alfalfa sprouts, tomatoes, asparagus, cabbage, cauliflower, spinach, and other green leafy vegetables. However, the chief source of vitamin K is synthesis by bacteria in the large intestine. This is a good reason to get the intestinal flora in good health so the liver can do its detoxification. Antioxidants are readily available in fresh fruits, especially citrus, and concentrated in fresh raw juices made from carrots, celery, beets, apples, and pears.

Alcohol

Alcohol is a challenging load for the liver and other parts of the digestive system. Alcohol inflames the lining of the stomach and can cause internal bleeding. Alcohol relaxes the lower esophageal sphincter, allowing stomach acids to flood the lower esophagus and induce heartburn. If a person is already suffering from diarrhea or nausea, even a moderate amount of alcohol will aggravate the symptoms. Heavy drinking over time is a leading cause of liver and pancreatic disease. Alcohol increases the possibilities of developing leaky gut syndrome, a condition where the mucous membrane is compromised and toxins and antigens enter the bloodstream.[27] It is rare to find a family that has not been touched by alcoholism.

Abstention or moderation, even extreme moderation, is recommended, because anything beyond a moderate amount of alcohol is bad for the health. Drinking only a moderate amount of alcohol can be difficult. Alcohol can so cloud the judgment that it may be difficult to define "moderate drinking." What does moderate drinking mean? The Mayo Clinic offers these guidelines: "No more than one drink a day for women or two drinks a day for men. A drink is defined as twelve ounces of beer, five ounces of wine, or one and a half ounces of 80 proof distilled spirits."[28] Think before you drink.

Gallbladder

The gallbladder is a small, bag-like organ lying just below the liver, where bile produced by the liver is concentrated and stored. The gallbladder passes bile into the duodenum. Bile breaks down molecules of cholesterol, fat, and fat-soluble vitamins into smaller globules, creating a larger surface area to interact with the fat-splitting enzyme lipase.

Bile is concentrated and thicker in the gallbladder than it is when it flows fresh from the liver. This thickening enables the three-inch-long gallbladder to store lots of the bile components. This concentration is susceptible to the formation of gallstones, an especially painful condition. These crystal-like grains of cholesterol or calcium salts cause excruciating pain and sudden projectile vomiting when they become lodged in the bile ducts entering the duodenum. While being overweight is a risk factor for gallstones, caution is urged when losing weight. Rapid or excessive weight loss can generate gallstone formation. Gradually losing weight at a rate of one to two pounds a week is less likely to instigate gallstone problems.[29]

Western medicine usually recommends the removal of a gallbladder filled with stones. Although gallbladder removal has become a routine procedure, many people are naturally hesitant about the surgical removal of body parts.

Fortunately some cases can be dealt with through dietary control, so why go in for avoidable surgery? I have had excellent results with reducing the symptoms of gallstones by limiting fats and oils. However, this course of action requires a consultation with a medical professional.

There is a gallbladder/liver cleanse promoted as a natural way to get rid of gallstones that I feel compelled to caution you about. Some folk remedies recommend heavy doses of pectin and malic acid from apples and other natural sources to soften the stones so they ostensibly can be passed without pain. Although there have been animal studies indicating that pectin can help dissolve gallstones, human successes are mostly anecdotal.[30]

A problem is possible when the "remedy" recommends drinking oil, usually olive oil, to "flush out" the stones. The idea is simple enough—the gallbladder, during the process of breaking down the oil, squirts bile through the bile duct and the pectin-reduced gallstones pass into the duodenum and out in the stool. Trouble may arise if the stones are too large or misshapen to pass through the narrow bile duct from the gallbladder to the duodenum. Extreme pain is a clear sign there is an emergency, and surgery is often the recommended treatment.

Pancreas

The pancreas is a six-inch-long organ resembling a stem thickly packed with ripe berries. The pancreas is primarily known for the production of the hormone insulin. The pancreas also produces enzyme-laden digestive juices that break down carbohydrates, proteins, and fats. These pancreatic enzymes are highly alkaline and neutralize the acidic chyme produced in the stomach.

The pancreatic enzymes enter the pancreatic duct that threads through the center of the pancreas and join with bile from the liver and gallbladder (see the pancreas illustration on page 47). Fresh bile from the liver moves toward the duodenum from the left and right hepatic ducts. Stored bile from the gallbladder passes through the cystic duct and merges with the fresh bile from the liver in the common bile duct. In most people the common bile duct and the pancreatic duct unite and enter the duodenum together. Sometimes there is an accessory duct leading from the pancreas and emptying through the common bile duct.

As with any complicated organ, things can go wrong. If the insulin regulation for blood sugar fails, people develop diabetes. Low secretion of pancreatic enzymes can lead to vitamin B_{12} nonabsorption and other nutritional deficiencies.

Inflammation of the pancreas, or pancreatitis, is a serious disorder. It can begin within 12–24 hours after a large meal or a bout of heavy drinking. An agonizing pain in the center of the upper abdomen is often the first sign of trouble. The pain, accompanied by vomiting, can be felt through to the back. Internal bleeding around the pancreas can cause bruises to show up on the abdomen. In severe cases there is fever.

About half the time people suffering from pancreatitis also have gallstones. The sudden onset of pancreatitis requires immediate hospitalization. X-rays and blood samples may be needed to establish a diagnosis. The blood work includes a look at pancreatic enzyme levels and other body chemicals. If a diagnosis of pancreatitis is established, it is likely the end of any consumption of alcohol for the patient.[31] For most people the attack of pancreatitis will pass and they recover; for others it can be life

The Pancreas

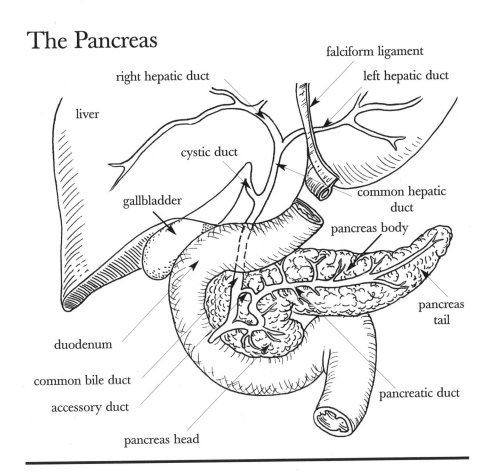

threatening. On occasion, blisters, called pseudocysts, form on the pancreas after an attack. Surgery may be required if this symptom occurs.

A number of studies have been done on the effects of alcohol, cigarette smoking, and coffee on pancreatitis. One study conducted at the Kaiser Permanente Medical Center in Oakland, California, found smoking to be an independent risk factor for pancreatitis that arises separately from drinking alcohol or from other unknown causes. The authors of the study speculated that smoking is either toxic to the pancreas or might give power to other toxins that affect the pancreas. The same study found that coffee drinking is associated with a reduced risk of pancreatitis. The suggested reason being that some ingredient in coffee may have a modulating effect on the pancreas of alcohol drinkers.[32]

Colon

The colon is the next vital section of the digestive tube. Chyme passes beyond the small intestine, through the ileocecal valve, and into one of nature's wonderful gifts—the large intestine—often unappreciated, hidden beneath a protruding abdomen, seen only as a tube of waste, filled with disease and sadness. We must look closer.

Like the small intestine, the three to eight feet of the colon are considered in portions. (See the illustration of the large intestine on page 49.) These are the ascending colon, running up the right side of the abdominal region; the transverse colon, traveling right to left from just beneath the lower forward points of the rib cage; and the descending colon, which follows. At the lower end of the descending colon is a horizontal twist called the sigmoid colon. The sigmoid colon is connected to the rectum and from there stool leaves the body. The tissues of the large intestine are fed by powerful streams of blood beating from the heart into the aorta and through a series of arteries. The large intestine passes potassium, water, sodium chloride, and the products of colonic bacteria—vitamin K, short-chain fatty acids, and volatile fatty acids—into the blood.

A vast complex of blood vessels, lymph vessels, and nerves surrounds the intestinal tract. A double layer of muscle wraps the intestine. The outer layer of muscle runs the length of the intestine, while the inner layer encircles the intestinal tube. In performing the work of mixing digestive juices and food moving the chyme along its path, the muscle layer gives form to the intestine. Inside the circular muscles are four layers of tissue: the submucosa, mucous membrane, the intestinal epithelium, and a coating of mucus. This interior interface is called the lumen.

The submucosa supports the mucous membrane between the circular muscles and the epithelium. The mucous membrane is speckled with mucus-secreting goblet cells. The thick layer of mucus from the goblet cells will smooth the way for food and fecal matter to move through the system and support friendly intestinal bacteria.

The Large Intestine

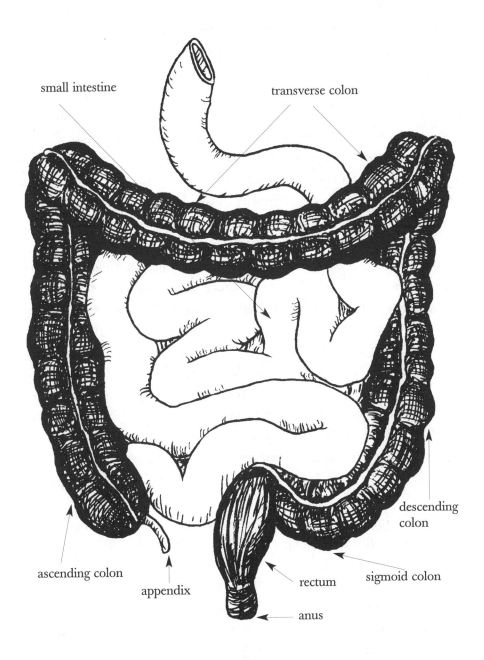

small intestine

transverse colon

ascending colon

appendix

rectum

anus

descending colon

sigmoid colon

Intestinal Flora

There is a world within our intestines composed of trillions of microorganisms. These are our gut microflora. They are as critical as the liver to cleansing health. The combined weight of the intestinal flora is about four pounds, just like the liver. Several ounces of new microbes are produced each day, while a similar amount is passed in the stool. Helpful bacteria are called probiotics; they guard against pathogens, synthesize vitamins, stimulate the immune system, and help to digest our food. The term "probiotics" is often used to describe supplements containing helpful bacteria, which are available in health food stores.

Over 400 species of one-celled organisms live in our intestinal tract. Bacterial cells in our intestines outnumber all other cells in our body ten to one.[33] The bacterial density increases in concentration the farther down the intestinal tract we look. Numbers can reach a trillion per milliliter of feces in the colon. The importance of this internal ecosystem to our health cannot be underestimated. Not all of these bacterial cells are friendly or neutral. Some bacteria produce toxins, generate immune reactions, and can even aid the growth of cancer cells. The numbers of harmful bacteria are held in check by the abundance of friendly bacteria. That is not the only role of friendly bacteria. They also digest our foods, producing vitamin K and the B vitamins—folic acid, biotin, pantothenic acid, and B_{12}. We feed the bacteria and the bacteria feed us. The absurd idea of a "self" separate from the rest of life is exposed by our reliance on intestinal bacteria. Without this healthy collection of relationships the individual dies.

A recently introduced method of keeping harmful bacteria, such as salmonella, out of the food supply is food irradiation. This is definitely helpful to the nuclear industry because it provides a "use" for nuclear wastes. Many researches are horrified for three principal reasons. One is the risk of handling nuclear materials at numerous irradiating facilities scattered across the country. Another problem is the loss of nutrients caused by irradiating foods; for example, milk loses most of its vitamin A, thiamin, and riboflavin when it is irradiated. The third and possibly most troubling reason to oppose irradiation is that it creates molecules in the food that are found nowhere else in nature. The FDA classes the molecules, which it calls radiolytic by-products, into two categories. One category is "known radiolytic products," which includes known carcinogens such as formaldehyde and benzene. The other is "unique radiolytic products" that have unknown effects.[34] Avoid irradiated foods.

The health of the intestinal microflora can be negatively affected by a variety of illnesses, dietary changes, and drug treatments—especially antibiotics. In some cases, where antibiotics destroy normal, health-promoting bacteria, there are life-threatening infections of *C. difficile* or other dangerous bacteria. It works like this: Beneficial bacteria, like *Lactobacillus acidophilus*, grow in such tight colonies on the intestinal wall that pathogenic microbes, viruses, and fungi have nowhere to take hold. Antibiotics destroy *Lactobacillus acidophilus* and the body experiences an overgrowth of dangerous bacteria, allowing chronic, systemic disease to set in. A common example for women is the onset of vaginal yeast infections after taking antibiotics.

When using probiotic supplements it is generally recommended to give *Bifidobacteria infantis* to toddlers and *Lactobacillus acidophilus* to adults. Consult with a health professional before giving probiotic supplements to toddlers. To make it through the upper digestive system and into the friendly parts of the lower intestine, probiotic supplements should be

NATURAL SOURCES OF PREBIOTICS

apples	citrus fruits	okra
asparagus	corn	onions
bananas	garlic	peas
barley	Jerusalem artichokes	rye
broccoli	kidney beans	soybeans
burdock root	leeks	summer squash
chicory	lentils	wheat
	oatmeal	

buffered with food and protection in the form of "prebiotics." Prebiotics are foods for friendly bacteria that pass undigested into the large intestine. Look for probiotic supplements with the prebiotics fructooligosaccharides (FOS) or inulin.[35] FOS and inulin are fibers known to increase beneficial bacteria in the colon. Natural sources of FOS and inulin are asparagus, fruit, garlic, leeks, maple syrup, onions, soybeans, and, in smaller amounts, whole rye and whole wheat.[36]

When the balance of the intestinal flora is disturbed by anything that reduces the friendly bacteria, disease-producing organisms such as candida, clostridium, *Hafnia alvei*, and citrobacter flourish in the microbial vacuum. Clostridium is a spore-forming, disease-causing, motile bacterium. *Hafnia alvei* causes infection and diarrhea by an unknown mechanism. Although *Citrobacter freundii* is found in a normal intestine, these and other species of citrobacter can cause a variety of diseases.

Lymph

The lymphatic system plays a major roll in removing toxic proteins, absorbing fats from food, and fighting infections.

The powerful beating of the heart creates such an intense fluid pressure in the capillaries that water, proteins, and other materials leak out. This leaked nutrient-rich liquid is called the interstitial fluid. The cells of the body are bathed and nourished by the interstitial fluid. Most of the interstitial fluid seeps back into the capillaries with low fluid pressure. The rest finds its way back into the bloodstream by a different route called the lymphatic system. When the interstitial fluid enters into the lymphatic system, it is called lymph. Lymph typically contains lymphocytes (T cells and B cells of the immune system), along with a wide range of waste from all parts of the body. Lymph comes from the blood and returns to the blood. Along its route are bean-shaped masses of tissue called lymph nodes. In the over 600 lymph nodes, waste, especially bacteria, are filtered out and prevented from entering the bloodstream, while lymphocytes are allowed to pass through.

When the lymph system is overloaded, the nodes can feel enlarged and tender. You can test yourself by using your fingers to press the nodes under your jaw, between the jaw and the ear, the groin area, the armpits, and the base of the skull. Tenderness indicates acute infection. Swollen nodes that are not tender indicate a chronic condition. Swollen lymph nodes can be indicators of serious diseases of the lymph system or even cancer. If you have persistent swollen lymph nodes, see a medical doctor.

The heartbeat does not circulate the lymph. Lymph is moved by muscular contraction. Any vigorous aerobic exercise, massage, deep diaphragmatic breathing, and yogic postures—especially twisting—will all help circulate the lymph.

THE LARGE INTESTINE:
Problems and Solutions

The large intestine provides important services for our health. Foremost it passes waste from all other organs of digestion. Poisons, cellular wastes, and most of the water that enters the digestive system is reabsorbed in the large intestine. Failure of the large intestine to reabsorb water results in diarrhea and dehydration. Additionally the large intestine absorbs sodium and other ions from the chyme. Intestinal bacteria produce vitamin K. Potassium, short-chain fatty acids, and volatile fatty acids pass from the large intestine into the blood. Numerous parasites can find a home in the large intestine. The intestine is vulnerable to great discomfort and disease from the materials passing through and from stress that originates elsewhere in the body. It is subjected to polyps and cancer. Fortunately there are steps that can be taken to alleviate most problems. An efficiently operating large intestine is a foundation for health.

Constipation

Constipation is the infrequent or difficult passage of hard, dry stools and is a source of extreme discomfort. Stool should pass without discomfort or strain. On completion of a successful bowel movement there should be no feeling of blockage or incomplete emptying. A good-looking stool should be brown, moist, somewhat cylindrical, with a point at one end. A lot can be learned by examining stool color. (See Dietary Causes of Stool Color, page 79, and Disease Causes of Stool Color, page 78.) If it has been in the colon for too long, stool comes out looking like little balls all pressed together. The pressure of passing hardened feces can cause hemorrhoids, varicose veins, rectal fissures, anal fissures, and pockets in the intestinal wall that can become dangerously infected. Constipation slows bowel activity—allowing proteins to putrefy, fats to grow rancid, and sugars to ferment. When we are constipated, toxins that are passing through the system have longer periods of contact with the intestinal walls. Bile acids concentrate in the constipated bowel, irritating the colon wall. Hormones the body is trying to pass are reabsorbed and alter hormonal balance.

There are many causes of constipation; often they have to do with stress, activity level, and/or what, when, and how much we eat and drink. Certain medications or medical conditions can cause constipation. Temporary constipation is often related to emotional stress, travel, or a change in diet. Long-term constipation can be the result of poor bathroom habits, improper diet, difficulties scheduling toilet time during work hours or at crowded facilities, and so forth.

Mild constipation will usually pass on its own. For most people the bowels will begin proper movement after a few days or a week.[1] The body knows best. Try taking advantage of the first 15 minutes after breakfast, a time of high colonic activity, to move the bowels or engage in bowel moving exercises, especially those done sitting on the toilet (see page 110). The bowels usually move best following meals.

Never ignore attacks of abdominal pain.

Causes of Constipation

acute appendicitis
anorexia nervosa
anthrax
autoimmune thyroid diseases
Behçet's disease
botulism food poisoning
bowel obstruction
bulimia nervosa
colorectal cancer
colorectal polyps
depression
diabetes insipidus
diabetic neuropathy
diverticular disease
Down syndrome
endometriosis
fecal impaction
food intolerances
Hashimoto's thyroiditis
headache-free migraine
Hirschsprung's disease
hyperparathyroidism
hypothyroidism
infant botulism food poisoning

intestinal obstruction
irritable bowel syndrome
lead poisoning
lichen sclerosus
megacolon
multiple myeloma
myxedema
obstipation
ovarian cancer
paralytic ileus
pernicious anemia
pheochromocytoma
porphyria
pregnancy
premenstrual syndrome
proctitis
Shy-Drager syndrome
small intestine cancer
stomach cancer
strongyloidiasis
thyroid disorders
typhoid fever
uterine prolapse
yellow fever

Medications

Most medications will have some effect on digestion. These effects can range from mild and unnoticeable, to constipation and internal bleeding. Many over-the-counter and prescription drugs create constipation as a side effect. Painkillers, such as those containing codeine and oxycodone, commonly cause constipation. Antispasmodics, antidepressants, and tranquilizers also contribute to the problem. Sometimes a physician may reduce the dosage or prescribe another drug in order to return the bowels to some normalcy.

Some of the most commonly used over-the-counter drugs, especially nonsteroidal anti-inflammatory drugs (NSAIDs), are among the most dangerous. Over 33 million Americans regularly take NSAIDs.[2] Worldwide, NSAIDs generate $5 billion in sales annually.[3] This group of generally effective medications includes aspirin, ibuprofen, naproxen, and ketoprofen, all sold under a variety of brand names. If they become a regular part of a person's self-treatment, or if used in excess of the recommended amount, they can cause stomach pain, ulcers, nausea, and diarrhea.[4]

Using capsule endoscopy, a pill-sized video camera swallowed by patients, researchers at Baylor College of Medicine viewed the small intestines of 41 adults who had been taking NSAIDs daily for three months to treat arthritis. Doctors found an astounding 71 percent of the patients in the study had ulcerations in their small intestines. Among 25 percent of the patients, the damage was deemed "severe."[5] Lead researcher Waqar Qureshi, MD, asserts, "NSAIDs weaken the protective barrier of the GI [gastrointestinal] tract, so that acids are more likely to cause damage."[6]

Although NSAIDs may provide temporary relief from pain, most NSAIDs can cause liver problems ranging from function test abnormalities due to a mild and reversible elevation of liver enzymes to severe hepatic necrosis.[7] This can cause an overload of bloodstream toxins, further aggravating the cycles of pain.

Consistent users of NSAIDs should see a health care provider to learn ways to limit the damage or find alternatives. Taking the lowest effective dose NSAIDs and taking them on a full stomach can mitigate damage. Acetaminophen is a non-NSAID pain reliever that might work in certain cases.

Other pain relievers, especially narcotics, can produce constipation. Blood pressure medications can cause diarrhea or constipation. Antibiotics can cause nausea or diarrhea while they are being taken. Additional problems can arise because the antibiotics destroy beneficial bacteria in the digestive system.

Disease and Constipation

There are occasions when constipation is the result of common disorders, such as diverticulitis, or more seriously, cancer. Disease is likely the culprit if adults who have previously experienced regular bowel movements begin to have a persistent change in character or frequency.

There have been two studies linking constipation and breast cancer. A study of over 7,000 women reported in the *American Journal of Public Health* showed an increase in breast cancer in women with constipation.[8] A study reported in the *Lancet* by physicians Nicholas L. Petrakis and Eileen B. King of the University of California, involving 1,500 women, showed that women having two bowel movements a week had four times the rate of breast cancer as women who had one or more daily bowel movements.[9] Additionally, Dr. Petrakis noted a few critical differences between the bowels of vegetarians and meat eaters. Meat eaters have greater amounts of mutagenic substances in their bowels and, perhaps more specific to breast cancer, certain species of intestinal bacterial flora that interfere with the linkages needed to complete the excretion of estrogen introduced to the gut in bile. It is theorized that some of the "unlinked" estrogen is reabsorbed in the large intestine of meat eaters, possibly leading to higher estrogen levels and the subsequent growth of cancers with estrogen receptors.[10]

Some naturopathic doctors assert that feces can harden and remain in the nooks and crannies of the large intestine for months and even years. The pioneering nutritionist and chiropractor Bernard Jensen reported seeing people who had expelled grape seeds but had not eaten grapes for nine months! "Where had those seeds been? I've seen popcorn come out of a person when they hadn't had popcorn for three years. Where had it been?" Dr. Jensen answers his question this way: "We accumulate these things in the mucous membrane that holds toxic material in various folds of the intestines."[11] Dr. Jensen believes that such residues are common. The whole grains advocate John Harvey Kellogg, MD, concurred, writing, "Of the 22,000 operations I have personally performed, I have never found a single normal colon."[12] Which begs the question—just what is "normal"?

The mechanics of constipation cause their own sets of problems. To force along the small hard lumps of stool the abdominal muscles contract, a deep breath is held, and the diaphragm is forced downward. Often the strain shows even in the muscles of the neck and face. The muscle strain used to pass difficult stools damages veins throughout the body—most especially creating hemorrhoids and varicose veins.[13]

Both hemorrhoids and varicose veins pop out when the interior valves of the veins are damaged or overridden by the pressure. Blood is pumped through the arteries by the electro-muscular contractions of the heart. Blood delivers oxygen and nutrients to the cells and returns to the heart through veins. Instead of surging, as it does through the arteries, the "used" blood in the veins is coaxed along and kept from flowing backwards by one-way valves located at intervals along the interior of the veins. When the valves are not working properly, blood backs up. The pressure is especially strong in the legs where, during the day, a four-foot-high column of blood exerts constant pressure on the veins. These veins stand out blue and raggedy, like the roads on a map of a pale, suffering land. Varicose veins are not only visually distracting—they can cause bouts of pain and lead to ulcers.

The mechanism is similar for hemorrhoids—the painful swelling of veins in the lower portions of the intestinal tract, the rectum, and the anus. Healthy veins here have two primary functions—not only do they return deoxygenated blood to the heart, they act as blood-filled cushions, preventing feces and gas from leaking out. Under the pressure of constipation, the veins will blow up like blood-filled balloons, painful and prone to infection.

It is possible to mistakenly believe a person is constipated. The hardness of the stool and not the frequency of the bowel movement is a primary indicator of constipation.[14] One question that generates an incredible range of strong opinions is how often the bowels are to be moved. Once a day is the standard held by many Americans. Others call for a movement after every meal, asking us to never say "no" to the urge. I'm inclined to agree with that.

Those advocating a loose standard of bowel movement frequency got a boost some decades ago when Walter C. Alvarez, MD, supervised an experiment where healthy, young medical students swallowed gelatin capsules filled with small glass beads. A few students passed nearly all the beads in the first 24 hours. Most students took four days to pass three-fourths of the beads. After nine days there were still some students who had passed only half the beads. Dr. Alvarez noted that the students who passed the most beads in 24 hours had loose stools containing undigested material. Those students with slower rates, who often believed they were constipated, had well-formed stools that showed evidence of good digestion. This experiment can lead many to the conclusion that a wide range of time may elapse between bowel movements without any impairment to our health. A person may have two or three bowel movements a day or have one every two or three days and still be in perfect health.[15]

If you like, you can perform an experiment similar to the one conducted by Dr. Alvarez. To discover the transit time of your food, eat a cup or two of red beets. Note the time they are eaten. The beets will color the stool quite dark, often reddish to purple. Just watch for the color change in the stool to see how long it takes for the passage. (Besides, beets are rich in phytonutrients and the antioxidant anthocyanidin.)[16]

Mind and Constipation

What is the first action we should take if we have constipation? Relax. Most instances of constipation will pass without worry or strain. The body can handle it.

It is important to create a relaxed and supportive toilet environment. My grandmother referred to moving the bowels as "doing your business." In this she appears to be intuitively in touch with one of the precepts of the ancient design principles of *feng shui*. Feng shui is a system of understanding originating in China perhaps 5,000 years ago. Literally translated, feng shui means "wind and water." Feng shui teaches that water is symbolic of business, wealth, and success. Water is central to the functions of the bathroom and toilet. It makes a difference when we put attention into the flow of positive energy in and around the bathroom. Water is regularly flushed from the bathroom, taking with it, well, we know what it takes with it. Feng shui practitioners recommend the bathroom be kept clean and uncluttered. They encourage the "yang" of warm colors and the soft light of candles to promote balance and positive energy in this mostly "yin" environment.[17]

A positive environment is conducive to clear thinking. German archaeologists have recently discovered the toilet of the Protestant reformer Martin Luther. The spacious 30 x 30-foot room was sheltered by a vaulted ceiling above a stone toilet.[18] Martin Luther called it the "secret place." It was there, during an extended bout of constipation, he wrote the Ninety-Five Theses that launched the Protestant Reformation.[19]

The feedback mechanisms between the bowels and the highest potentials of the mind are so closely related that ayurvedic teacher Harish Johari considers care of the bowels to be preparation for spiritual practice. "Meditation can only be done when the stomach is clear and clean, when there are no toxins in the body. No meditation is possible if you have not been to the toilet."[20] The late Swami Vishnudevananda agreed, saying, "Purity of the mind is not possible without purity of the body in which it functions, and by which it is affected."[21]

Many times constipation in adults can be traced to problems that arose when they first received toilet training as children. In *Dr. Spock's Baby and Child Care* (8th edition) there is a summary of the philosophy and methods of toilet training endorsed by pediatrician T. Berry Brazelton.[22] The text argues against using force, coercion, or criticism when toilet training children. Dr. Brazelton's cases revealed that children trained in this way were the least likely to develop problems with bed-wetting and daytime soiling. Parents are encouraged to use tactful suggestions and flattery so children get a clear understanding that eventual success is expected. Parents should give mild praise and encouragement when a child is successful. Patience is required of parents. Anger and criticism have no place in toilet training.[23]

In what other ways does poor training create problems later in life? When the urge to move the bowels is ignored, the sensation will pass. The addition of more food into the system will renew the urge. Consistent efforts to ignore the messages of the body will cause the rectum to eventually fail to signal. The resulting constipation can be severe.

Sometimes a large, hard stool can result in hemorrhoids or tear a tiny slit or fissure at the edge of the stretched anus. These can be quite painful. Bowel movements that follow can reopen the wound. This can cause children to fear going to the toilet, generating more constipation and more painful movements. These painful conditions can cause even adults to further suppress the urge to defecate. A change in diet or a physician-recommended stool softener may be appropriate in these cases.

Some of the problems can arise when symptoms of a more serious ailment are diagnosed incorrectly. Pain is seldom associated with constipation. Assuming that abdominal pain is caused by constipation can lead to people dosing themselves with laxatives when the source of their pain may be something more severe, such as a ruptured appendix with peritonitis, requiring immediate medical attention. Abdominal pain can also be caused by intestinal spasms that are perceived as abdominal cramps. Intestinal spasms often can be traced to emotional distress. Constipation may be associated with acute illnesses, old age, medications, or even simple cases of prolonged inactivity, poor food choices, or dehydration.

Laxatives

There are times when a mild laxative might be beneficial, however there are real drawbacks. Consumer Union's *The Medicine Show* notes, "There can be no doubt that laxatives have contributed more to the ills and discomforts of mankind than the condition they are supposed to relieve."[24] To purge the bowels when fluid reserves are already depleted can be disastrous. There are no perfect commercial products to alleviate constipation, and yet the laxative industry today boasts a cash flow of hundreds of million of dollars a year.

The body of any individual may react more or less strongly to a laxative. A laxative for one is a cathartic for another. The same person may react differently to the same dosage at different times. If you use a laxative, it is wise to use the least amount of the most gentle laxative that works.

When laxatives are employed to end constipation, a cycle of degenerating health may begin. Although the constipation that first inspires the use of laxatives can arise from myriad causes, continued use of laxatives brings changes in both the muscle tone and lining of the bowel. Extended use of laxatives can cause the natural muscular reflexes to become diminished, requiring stronger and stronger doses of the laxative to move the bowels. Regular use of certain laxatives can deplete the body's supply of potassium, further weakening the muscles.

After years of taking laxatives, the colon may be stretched into twisted coils that loop around to twice their original length. In those cases it may take days to fill the colon enough to stimulate a bowel movement.[25]

Prunes, prune extract, and prune juice are wonderful ways to promote the contraction and relaxation of the intestines, propelling the contents along and ending constipation. Prunes are rich sources of fiber, vitamin A, and potassium. Potassium draws water into the fecal matter making it softer and easier to move.

The visionary physician John McDougall recommends, as a last resort for constipation, a nonabsorbable prescription sugar called lactulose. According to Dr. McDougall, lactulose draws water into the colon and helps to end constipation in even the toughest cases.[26]

Fiber is critical in maintaining regular bowel movements. Including high-fiber foods as a regular part of the diet will go a long way toward warding off constipation. There are fiber supplements that should be taken with plenty of water. Some supplements are mostly bran; others, such as Citrucel, contain methylcellulose, and Metamucil uses psyllium. (For a more detailed discussion of fiber see Fiber and Carbohydrates, pages 17-22. Fiber and colon cancer are discussed on pages 83-84.) Some folks get temporary relief from constipation with magnesium-containing laxatives such as milk of magnesia and magnesium citrate. Magnesium-containing laxatives can cause magnesium and sodium overload in older adults with renal dysfunction.

Enemas

Enemas can be effective for some people as an alternative to laxatives. Thousands of years ago Egyptians had an advanced understanding of the bowels, which grew out of their attempts to preserve the body after death. The embalmers noted the bacterial putrefaction of the intestines of the corpse. This led them to remove the intestines and stomach as a part of the mummification process.[27] They came to associate feces with decay; as a result, they made liberal use of enemas and laxatives among the living.[28] Written instructions for the use of enemas are found in the Edwin Smith Papyrus from around 1700 BCE and the Elbers Papyrus in the 14th century BCE.[29]

A common and safe enema consists of a pint of tepid water introduced to the last eight inches of the colon. This can clean out old, hardened feces and get them moving. Enemas can create problems if used too frequently. Even once a week will be too much for some people. The problem, as with laxatives, is that the bowels will stop moving without the new stimulation.[30]

Colonic Irrigation

Enemas should be distinguished from colonic irrigation, also known as colon hydrotherapy, a procedure where the large intestine is pressure-infused with water or other liquids that are introduced through the rectum. Colonic irrigation attempts to reach far beyond the first few inches of the colon flushed by an ordinary enema. "High colonic" is a loose term for colon hydrotherapy, flushing the large intestine with 20 or more gallons of liquid administered by a pump or gravity-fed device.[31] The United States Food and Drug Administration approves colonic irrigation systems as Class III devices to be used in medically indicated colon cleansing. The FDA specifically mentions, "such as before radiological or endoscopic examination."[32] Of course, even when specialists perform colon cleansing there is a risk of bowel perforation, especially in the elderly.[33] Adequate colonic cleansing is essential for accurate and safe colonic medical procedures. However, the use of colonic irrigation systems for general health improvement has not been sanctioned.[34]

I have heard many first person accounts of the benefits of colonic irrigation for general health and as a cure for numerous ailments. Nonetheless, I have my doubts and do not recommend this method of bowel cleansing.

Current mainstream medical understanding in the Western world is in general agreement: colonic irrigation for health improvement is not only useless but also dangerous.[35] Still, there are many advocates of colonic irrigation. In a recent article in the *Journal of Clinical Gastroenterology*, E. Ernst charges that "ignorance is celebrating a triumph over science." The article continues, "Today we are witnessing a resurgence of colonic irrigation based on little less than the old bogus claims and the impressive power of vested interests. Even today's experts on colonic irrigation can only provide theories and anecdotes in its support."[36]

Some of the most outstanding anecdotal support for colonic irrigation can be seen in the photographs offered in Dr. Jensen's books *Dr. Jensen's Guide to Better Bowel Care* and *Tissue Cleansing Through Bowel Management*. Not for the squeamish, each picture displays dark, rubbery-looking goop that has been expelled by patients using his system. Dr. Jensen's "Ultimate Cleansing Program" includes intestinal bulk, mostly fiber, mixed with clay and water and taken five times a day, followed by colonic irrigation.[37] Stephen Barrett, MD, an anti-colonic activist, believes much of the material expelled from the rectum and believed by colonic irrigation advocates to be feces accumulation is in fact "casts" formed by the fiber and clay the patients most recently ingested.[38]

A French investigation of the effects of bowel cleansing on the peristaltic action of the intestines was published in *Gut* magazine. Healthy subjects were tested. The study found no significant difference in the motility of the bowels after one month between those who had bowel cleansing and those who had not.[39]

The Consumer Union's book *The Medicine Show* cautions: "High colonic enemas are antiquated, useless, and sometimes harmful. They do not cure habitual constipation or remove 'toxins,' and in general do not promote health or prolong life."[40] The National Council Against Health

Fraud, a nonprofit, voluntary health agency, warns: "Consumers should not use colonics, and should avoid patronizing practitioners who employ this procedure. Practitioners who use colonics are either too ignorant or misguided to be entrusted with delivering health services."[41] The Infectious Disease Branch of the California Department of Health Services states: "Neither physicians nor chiropractors should be performing colonic irrigations. We are not aware of any scientifically proven health benefit of this procedure, yet we are well aware of its hazards."[42]

The hazards of colonic irrigation include the danger of excessive fluid absorption, perforation of the bowel, and fatal infection. Several outbreaks of serious infections have been reported from inadequately sterilized equipment. In one particularly nasty case, contaminated equipment caused amebiasis in 36 patients. Six of those patients also had perforated bowels. All of them died as a result.[43] I encourage you to make up your own mind about this controversial procedure.

Diarrhea

Diarrhea is a condition of loose, watery stools. A proper diagnosis from a trusted health care professional is essential if diarrhea lasts longer than one day or if there is fever, severe abdominal pains, or bloody stool. Although most viral attacks of diarrhea run their course in a couple days, some may last more than a week. There are many causes of diarrhea, including the use of antibiotics or other medications. Even doses of vitamin C can promote diarrhea. Diarrhea may be a symptom of more serious conditions, such as amoebic dysentery or ulcerative colitis.

Diarrhea can even occur when the bowel becomes impacted with feces. Impacted feces in the bowel is usually thought of as a form of constipation; however with some conditions, such as irritable bowel syndrome, the body may liquefy the contents of the colon so that it passes through the compacted feces.[44]

The treatment of diarrhea depends on its cause. A danger of diarrhea, regardless of its source, is dehydration. Fluid loss from diarrhea should be offset by drinking plenty of liquids. There are times when prescription drugs may be the best way to treat acute diarrhea.

CAUSES OF DIARRHEA

acute appendicitis
acute kidney failure
Addisonian crisis
Addison's disease
allergies
anaphylaxis
anthrax
autonomic neuropathy
Behçet's disease
Blastocystis hominis
bowel obstruction
Brainerd diarrhea
celiac disease
chemical pneumonia
cholera
ciguatera poisoning
classic galactosemia
Clostridium perfringens
colitis
colorectal cancer
colorectal polyps
common migraine
constipation (small,
    dry, hard feces
    alternating with
    diarrhea)
Crohn's disease
cryptosporiosis
cyclic vomiting
    syndrome
cyclosporiasis
cystic fibrosis (foul-
    smelling, greasy,
    bulky, mucus)
diabetes insipidus
diabetic diarrhea
diabetic neuropathy

diarrheagenic
    Escherichia coli
Dientamoeba fragilis
diverticular disease
Ebola
E. coli food poisoning
ehrlichiosis
endometriosis
Entamoeba histolytica
enteritis
enterocolitis
enterotoxigenic
    Escherichia coli
Escherichia coli
    O157:H7
fascioliasis
favism
fecal impaction
fecal incontinence
food allergies
food intolerances
food poisoning
gastrinoma
gastritis
gastroenteritis
gastrointestinal
    anthrax
giardia
glanders
headache-free
    migraine
hemolytic uremic
    syndrome
hepatitis
Hirschsprung's disease
HIV/AIDS
hookworm
hyper-IgM syndrome

hyperthyroidism
inflammatory bowel
    disease
intestinal pseudo-
    obstruction
irritable bowel
    syndrome
lactose intolerance
Lassa fever
Legionnaires' disease
leptospirosis
listeriosis
malabsorption
Marburg virus
mastocytosis
melioidosis
Ménétrier's disease
meningitis
middle ear infection
multiple endocrine
    neoplasia type 1
mycobacterium avium
    complex
neuroblastoma
Norwalk-like viruses
ovarian cancer
pellagra
pernicious anemia
radiation sickness
rapid gastric emptying
Reiter's syndrome
Rocky Mountain
    spotted fever
rotavirus
Salmonella enteritis
salmonella food
    poisoning
SARS

schistosomiasis	stomach cancer	viral dysentery
SCID	strongyloidiasis	viral gastroenteritis
scombrotoxic fish poisoning	toxic shock syndrome	viral hepatitis
	traveler's diarrhea	viral meningitis
short bowel syndrome	trichinosis	Weil's syndrome
Sjögren's syndrome	typhoid fever	Whipple's disease
sprue	ulcerative colitis	whipworm
Staphylococcus aureus (food poisoning)	urinary tract infections	whooping cough
		yersiniosis
steatorrhea (foul-smelling)	*Vibrio parahaemolyticus*	Zollinger-Ellison syndrome
	Vibrio vulnificus	

Irritable Bowel Syndrome

Irritable bowel syndrome (IBS) is a disease that can affect nearly every part of the gastrointestinal tract. Irritable bowel syndrome is characterized by abnormal muscular contractions, especially a spastic colon, sometimes resulting in alternating constipation and bouts of diarrhea. The stool is likely to have excessive mucus. IBS is often associated with abdominal cramping, gas, bloating, and even a crampy urge to defecate without the bowels being moved. We do not know the causes of IBS and there is no certain cure. No sign of disease can be seen in the colon of a person suffering from irritable bowel syndrome, placing the disease in the category of functional disorders, where physiological functions are altered rather than an identifiable structural or biochemical cause. Although IBS is a serious cause of distress in and of itself, there is no evidence that it causes bleeding or permanent harm to the intestines.

The muscles that control contraction and relaxation (peristalsis) of the colon in people with irritable bowel syndrome seem to be extremely sensitive and reactive. This sensitivity causes the muscles to spasm in the presence of stimulation that would not bother most people. IBS symptoms can be triggered by gas, medications, particular foods, or even the simple act of eating. If medications and certain foods set the IBS symptoms in motion, they should be noted and avoided. Eating normally stimulates the peristaltic action, but in irritable bowel syndrome the reaction is exaggerated.

Emotions can trigger IBS symptoms, disrupting normal peristalsis and bringing on abdominal pain, distention, explosions of gas, and hard stools alternating with loose stools. The majority of people with irritable bowel syndrome who go to a gastrointestinal specialist are also dealing with some kind of emotional problem.[45] Irritable bowel syndrome itself can be a significant source of emotional distress. When there appears to be an emotional component to IBS symptoms, it is important to at least cushion the anxiety and stress.

There are other causes of the symptoms normally found with IBS. So a diagnosis of IBS should not be assumed until the possibility of other conditions or diseases have been eliminated. For some the cause may be food intolerance. Some people lack the intestinal enzyme lactase that is required to digest cow's milk and foods made from it. Other foods may cause episodes of similar discomfort.

There are ways to treat and manage the symptoms of irritable bowel syndrome. Relief can come from medications, dietary adjustments, and stress management. There may be times when lifestyle adjustments and dietary modifications will not be enough to control IBS symptoms. Your doctor or health care provider may recommend fiber supplements and/or medications to reduce cramps, spasms, and diarrhea.

To help monitor food intake, the University of Pittsburgh Medical Center (UPMC) recommends keeping a food diary where a list of what foods are eaten, when they are eaten, and the body's reactions (if any) are recorded. UPMC encourages discussing the food diary results with a doctor or dietician and making gradual dietary changes. The recommendation is to avoid foods that trigger symptoms more than once.[46]

Eat plenty of fiber, increasing the amounts gradually. Too much too soon can increase gas and bloating until the body adjusts. Painful spasms may be reduced by the mild distention of the colon caused by the fiber. The increased water retention of the fiber keeps stools soft and less painful to pass. Fiber can be supplemented by a gradual increase of fruits,

DIARRHEA

Contact a health professional if diarrhea lasts longer
than one day or is accompanied by: (1) a fever
(2) severe abdominal pain (3) bloody stool

vegetables, nuts, and whole grains. Brown rice is a nearly perfect food, as it is a whole grain high in fiber.

Eating too much food at one sitting can trigger IBS symptoms. Eat five or six smaller meals throughout the day instead of the more traditional three large meals. Eat smaller portions. Do not gobble food. Go slowly, and try to avoid swallowing air. Drinking lots of water can reduce constipation.

The colon is tied to the brain by powerful nerves. Emotional stress can set off IBS. Energy being used for emotional stress is not available for healing. Stress reduction can involve a wide variety of techniques, such as biofeedback, counseling, and exercise.

Exercise has the advantage of both reducing stress and improving bowel function. The McKinley Health Center at the University of Illinois lists exercise as a critical treatment for IBS, noting on their Web site: "[Exercise] helps relieve the symptoms of anxiety and also promotes good bowel function."[47] Be sure to consult with a health care professional before beginning any exercise program.

Hatha yoga exercises and postures have been used for generations for relaxation, health, and spiritual awareness. Those new to yoga practice should seek out an experienced teacher and adapt the exercises to their personal abilities, suppleness, and physical constitution.

There is mounting and compelling evidence that hypnotherapy is an effective treatment for irritable bowel syndrome.[48] Olafur S. Palsson, PsyD, reviews over a dozen published research studies on hypnosis for irritable bowel syndrome at www.ibshypnosis.com. British researchers found that three months of hypnotherapy could relieve symptoms and maintain that relief for more than five years after the cessation of treatment.[49]

Irritable bowel syndrome is common, and there are numerous sources that provide an in-depth analysis of it. More general information for the treatment of irritable bowel syndrome may be found at the International Foundation for Functional Gastrointestinal Disorders (IFFGD), 1-888-964-2001, www.iffgd.org.

Leaky Gut Syndrome

Leaky gut syndrome is the condition of increased permeability of the intestinal wall due to loss of the mucous membrane, or where the cells or spaces between the cells are compromised, permitting toxins and antigens to pass into the bloodstream. There are a number of causes of leaky gut syndrome, most of them having to do with the destruction of friendly bacteria and the overgrowth of disease-causing bacteria. The imbalance of the intestinal flora can create inflammation and injury to the protective membrane, opening the way to leaky gut syndrome.

Antibiotics, including colloidal silver, pose the danger of intestinal flora disruption. Eating lots of refined sugar and sugar-containing products boosts the growth of harmful microorganisms such as *Candida albicans*.[50] High-fiber foods protect the gut wall by feeding friendly aerobic bacteria.[51]

Problems with the intestinal wall and the bacteria enclosed within it play a complex role in the development of food sensitivity. Food sensitivity is an adverse reaction to a food, an additive, or another ingredient. Antigens are substances that induce a state of food sensitivity or an immune responsiveness. The presence of toxins and antigens increases the burdens on the liver and other parts of the immune system.

FOODS TO AVOID
caffeine
alcohol
high-fat foods
spicy foods
dairy products
onions
cabbage

Food intolerance is when the body reacts negatively to certain foods. Food intolerance usually involves the digestive system and is marked by an adverse reaction when a particular food or ingredient is consumed.

Interspaced in the lining of the intestine are immune system cells. When the immune system cells allow a substance to pass without reacting, it is called oral tolerance. Some food proteins or disease-causing bacteria stimulate the immune cells to react defensively. This reaction is called an allergic response. Allergies are immune system reactions to specific foods or something in those foods. The immune system treats the food item as an invasive toxin.

Alcohol consumption is a real danger. Even in amounts otherwise considered "moderate," alcohol can damage the intestinal membrane and encourage the overgrowth of harmful bacteria. Even healthy people have shown an increase in intestinal permeability after one shot of whisky.[52] Worse yet, consuming alcohol and an allergen at the same time can intensify the allergic reaction.

There are other causes of leaky gut syndrome that are not clearly related to harmful bacteria. For example, chemotherapy used to destroy fast-growing cancer cells can increase the permeability of the intestinal wall. Treating cancers located on or near the intestines with radiation can also damage the intestinal wall.

Parasites

Besides the beneficial and harmful intestinal flora, humans are also subjected to a number of worm-like parasites that can infect the human digestive tract. These multicellular, legless wigglers are known as metazoa, helminths, or worms. Among the most common and persistent are roundworms, tapeworms, whipworms, and schistosomiasis. The Centers for Disease Control recommend having a laboratory look for parasites or their eggs in three or more stool samples, collected on separate days, in order to have a high degree of diagnostic certainty.[53]

A type of roundworm, *Ascaris lumbricoides*, currently infects 1.5 billion people.[54] I have had personal experience with roundworms, although I didn't know it until the rubbery, foot-long adults started showing up in my stool. Roundworm eggs can get into the mouth from fingers that have touched contaminated soil. The eggs can even rise in dry dust and enter the nose or mouth with the breath. The adult worms live in the small intestines, sometimes filling much of the space. Ascaris larvae travel via the bloodstream and enter the lungs. They move up the throat to the pharynx, only to be swallowed and passed back to the small intestine where adult growth is completed. A mild ascaris infection might not bother some folks, but the adult worms can migrate to various parts of the body with serious effects.

Whipworm, another type of roundworm, causes infection throughout the world. At any given moment one billion people are infected with whipworm.[55] Small, blood-streaked, diarrhea-like stools, tenderness or pain in the abdomen, and sometimes severe anemia are symptoms of heavy whipworm infection. Strangely, University of Iowa researchers have reported preliminary evidence that swallowing whipworm eggs can cause a temporary harmless infection that may soothe inflammatory bowel disease by diverting the "attention" of the overactive immune reaction that can cause inflammatory bowel disease.[56]

Tapeworms, another parasite fond of humans, enter the body as eggs in undercooked beef, pork, or fish. The adult tapeworm attaches its small head to the wall of the large intestine. Pieces of the worm may show up in the stool, but unless the head is destroyed or passed the tapeworm persists. Beef and pork tapeworms can cause a variety of abdominal complaints. Fish tapeworms can create an anemia similar to pernicious anemia. If you feel you must eat meat, be sure it is well cooked to prevent tapeworm infection.

Intestinal schistosomiasis is contracted by contact with freshwater containing the free-swimming form of the parasite. It enters the human body by hooking into the skin and passing through it into the bloodstream. Drinking contaminated water gives access through the lining of the throat or esophagus. Adult worms can be found in the intestines, bladder, or other organs. Freshwater snails are host to this parasite in tropical waters from the Nile to Vietnam, currently infecting 265 million people.[57]

Giardia

Giardia lamblia is a one-celled, microscopic parasite that lives in the intestine and is passed in the stool. Giardia infection is highly contagious. It is probably the most common cause of parasitic gastrointestinal disease, infecting up to 20 percent of the world's population. In the United Sates alone up to 2.5 million cases of giardiasis occur each year.[58] Diarrhea leading to weight loss and dehydration can be caused by giardia, but not every infected person shows symptoms. Symptoms normally begin one to two weeks after ingestion and include diarrhea, flatulence, upset stomach, cramps, and nausea. Giardia stools tend to be greasy floaters, sometimes coming out green or pale in color. In healthy people, symptoms may last two to six weeks. Giardia is difficult to diagnose and may require a laboratory examination of a series of stool specimens over several days.

There are two forms of *Giardia lamblia*: an active form called a trophozoite, and an inactive form called a cyst. The trophozoite causes the signs and symptoms of giardiasis by attaching itself to the lining of the small intestine. The trophozoite cannot live long outside of the body; therefore it cannot spread the infection to others. The inactive cyst is protected by an outer shell that enables it to survive in the environment outside the body for extended periods of time. Infected people and animals can release millions of giardia cysts in a single bowel movement. Giardiasis can be caused by as few as ten cysts. Once giardia-contaminated food or drink are swallowed, the stomach acid activates the cyst, which then develops into the disease-causing trophozoite. Trophozoites produce new cysts that pass in the feces and spread the infection to others.

Giardia lamblia is one of the most common causes of waterborne disease in both drinking and recreational water in the United States. Giardia shows up in soil, food, water, and feces-contaminated surfaces. Infection occurs after swallowing the parasite in food that has come into contact with the feces of a person or animal infected with giardia. Getting water in the mouth from contaminated swimming pools, natural bodies of water, hot tubs, and Jacuzzis can transmit giardia. Contaminated food that is eaten raw or undercooked can spread the disease.

It is best to avoid giardia altogether. If you do get infected, several prescription drugs are available to treat giardia. Young children and pregnant women are especially susceptible to dehydration resulting from giardia-induced diarrhea and need to drink plenty of fluids while ill.

Shigella

Shigellosis is an infectious disease caused by the shigella bacteria. Common effects of shigella start a day or two after exposure and can include fever, stomach cramps, and bloody diarrhea. Young children and the elderly are especially vulnerable to the severe effects of the diarrhea and may require hospitalization. A severe infection in children under two years old can develop into a high fever with associated seizures. Shigellosis usually passes within five to seven days. Although some infected people may have no symptoms at all, they can still pass shigella bacteria to others. Even those with a shigella infection that causes intense diarrhea usually recover completely, although it may take several months for their bowels to return to normal.

About 18,000 cases of shigellosis are reported each year in the United States (more often in summer than winter). Milder cases are often not diagnosed or reported, so the actual number of infections may be 20 times greater.[59]

Laboratory tests of the stool of an infected person are required to identify shigella. Testing for shigella can be overlooked unless the lab receives specific instructions. Special tests are required to tell which kind of shigella the person has and what treatment might be appropriate.

Antibiotics may be recommended to kill the shigella bacteria in the patient's stools and shorten their illness. The most common antibiotics used are ampicillin, trimethoprim/sulfamethoxazole, ciprofloxacin, or nalidixic acid. Some shigella, like other bacteria, have evolved resistance to specific antibiotics. Using antibiotics to treat shigellosis can generate more resistant strains. For this reason it may be recommended that people with mild infections not take antibiotics. They will usually quickly recover without antibiotic treatment. The National Center for Infectious Diseases at the Centers for Disease Control and Prevention warns, "Antidiarrheal agents such as loperamide (Imodium) or diphenoxylate with atropine (Lomotil) are likely to make the illness worse and should be avoided."[60]

There are several types of shigella. Someone who has had a specific type of shigella is not likely to suffer a bad response to that type again for at least several years. Unfortunately, one type of shigella, *Shigella flexneri*, will cause about 3 percent of those genetically predisposed to develop Reiter's syndrome, which causes pain in the joints, irritation of the eyes, and painful urination. Reiter's syndrome can last for years and lead to chronic arthritis.

Infected people have shigella bacteria in their diarrhea stools while they are sick and for a week or two afterwards. Shigella infections pass from the stools or soiled fingers of one person to the mouth of another person. Toddlers who are not fully toilet trained are most likely to ingest shigella and spread it to family members and play-mates. Additionally, shigella infections can come from eating food contaminated by infected food handlers who have not washed their hands with soap after using the toilet. Flies breed in infected feces and then contaminate vegetables in fields and kitchens. Contaminated water can spread shigella to swimmers and drinkers.

Guidelines

The guidelines to avoid getting or spreading feces-borne diseases like giardia and shigella involve practicing good hygiene. Wash hands thoroughly with soap and water, especially before eating or preparing food, after using the toilet, and after changing diapers. If you work with children in diapers, even if you are wearing gloves, wash after each diaper change. Dispose of or wash soiled diapers properly, disinfect diaper-changing areas, and keep children with diarrhea from coming in contact with other kids. Make sure toddlers and small children do a good job of washing their hands after they use the toilet. Warn kids against drinking pool water.

Avoid water that might be contaminated. Do not drink untreated water. Do not swim in places such as pools, hot tubs, lakes, rivers, and the ocean in areas with giardia outbreaks. Infected people should not swim in these places for weeks after their diarrhea stops. Giardia can pass in the stool and contaminate water for several weeks after symptoms have ended.

Disease Causes of Stool Color

Red: blood in stool, usually lower GI bleeds from the colon, rectum, or anus; or very brisk and serious upper GI bleeds such as hemorrhagic ulcers, etc.

amoebic dysentery

anal fissure

bowel obstruction
   (blood-stained mucus)

cirrhosis of the liver

colitis

colorectal cancer

colorectal polyps

diverticular disease

dysentery

esophageal varices

food allergies

food poisoning

gastritis

gastrointestinal bleeding

glomerular disease

hemolytic uremic syndrome

hemorrhoids

hookworm

intestinal obstruction
   (blood-stained mucus)

peptic ulcer

portal hypertension

proctitis

rectal prolapse

schistosomiasis

shigellosis

small intestine cancer

stomach cancer

thrombocytopenia

tuberculosis

ulcerative colitis

Black: usually upper GI bleeds

gastric erosion

gastritis

gastrointestinal bleeding

hookworm

peptic ulcer

small intestine cancer

stomach cancer

thrombocytopenia

Clay-colored

gallstones

hepatitis

Greenish

giardia

salmonella

Pale Stool

celiac disease

cholangitis

cholecystitis

giardia

hepatitis

sprue

steatorrhea

viral hepatitis

Dietary Causes of Stool Color

black	asprin
	black licorice
	blueberries
	dark foods (such as chocolate sandwich cookies)
	iron rich foods (such as spinich)
	iron supplements
	Pepto-Bismol (bismuth)
green	food coloring as in green popsicles
	leafy green vegetables
	iron supplements
orange	beta-carotene supplements
	carrots
	sweet potatoes
	food colorings
pale or clay-colored	
	Kaopectate
	other antidiarrheal medications
	baruim
red or pink	beets
	red food coloring as in popsicles
	tomato juice or soup
yellow	gluten protein

Avoid untreated ice or drinking water when traveling in countries where the water supply might be not be safe. Be very careful of eating uncooked foods when traveling in countries with minimal water treatment and poor sanitation systems. Any food that is to be eaten raw should be washed in uncontaminated water. If the safety of the water supply is uncertain, peel all raw vegetables and fruits before eating them. Avoid foods and beverages that might be contaminated.

Polyps and Colon Cancer

Colorectal cancer, commonly called simply "colon cancer," is the third most frequent cancer in the United States with approximately 150,000 new cases occurring annually, leading to about 57,000 deaths each year.[61] Factors such as age, family history, obesity, diet, and lifestyle can all be significant risk factors for colon cancer.

Intestinal polyps are abnormal growths in the large intestine that can develop into colon cancer. The Calcium Polyp Prevention Study reveals the need for good supplies of both calcium and vitamin D to discourage the growth of polyps.[62] Earlier research had shown calcium and vitamin D independently provided protection against the growth of polyps, but the subsequent four-year randomized trial conducted through the Norris Cotton Cancer Center found that people deficient in calcium or vitamin D did not receive the benefits of either nutrient.[63] *Prevention* magazine recommends a daily supplemental dose of 100 percent of the daily value for vitamin D.[64] Calcium is best obtained through calcium-rich foods.

Inflammation

There is growing evidence of a direct link between inflammation and colon cancers.[65] How is it that inflammation might cause colon cancer? The answer to this question comes from the confluence of two streams of cancer investigation. The renowned pathologist Rudolf Virchow made the earliest speculation in the 1860s that cancer arises at the site of chronic inflammation. A hundred years later oncologists were noting the role genetic mutations play in aiding the abnormal growths that become cancer. The possibility is now being investigated that these two processes—inflammation and genetic mutation—combine to turn healthy cells into malignant tumors.[66]

When faced with an infection, large cells called macrophages mount part of the body's defense. The macrophages release cytokines—chemicals that induce more immune cells to flood the site of the infection. The immune cells not only destroy the pathogens, they also take out damaged tissue. One way the macrophages and other immune cells do this is by releasing highly reactive oxygen free radicals that can also destroy or damage DNA. If the DNA is destroyed, that is the end of it.[67] But if the DNA in a cell is only damaged, the cell may continue growing and dividing. This cell is abnormal but not necessarily cancerous.[68]

Unfortunately, the immune system may treat the abnormal cell like a wound. Some cancer biologists assert that proteins and growth factors are brought in, flooding the abnormal cells with nutrients. This could cause the cells to develop into a tumor.[69]

Some of these inflammatory cycles are well documented, such as the continual bathing of the esophagus with stomach acid, the condition known as chronic heartburn that predisposes people to esophageal cancer. Inflammation is one way the body removes toxins by killing off germs. Inflammation can also cause toxins to be diluted. The trick is to allow inflammation to do its work without causing damage.[70]

Aspirin (acetylsalicylic acid) is one of the mildest ways of treating inflammation. Willow trees produce salicytates—the basic substances from which acetylsalicylic acid is derived. Native Americans long used willow bark to reduce fever. The Hottentots of South Africa prepared a similar medicine for rheumatism. Hippocrates, the father of modern medicine, advocated chewing willow bark or leaves for fever relief in childbirth.[71]

The German chemist Felix Hofmann developed the modern compound sold as aspirin. Hofmann was troubled by the suffering of his father, who was crippled with the inflammation of rheumatism. His experiments developed into a commercial method for producing acetylsalicylic acid. Friedrich Bayer & Company put a powdered aspirin on the market in 1899.[72] The rest, as they say, is history.

The drug company Pfizer produced the anti-inflammatory drug Celebrex to treat the inflammation of arthritis. In 2000 researchers discovered that patients taking Celebrex for arthritis were less likely to develop intestinal polyps.[73] Similar results have been found with the millions of Americans taking the anti-inflammatory aspirin to prevent heart attacks. Evidence from Dartmouth Medical School researchers shows aspirin also fights colon cancer.[74] Celebrex and aspirin both block an enzyme produced during inflammation called cyclo-oxygenase 2 (COX-2). There is a possibility that COX-2 may trigger the development of precancerous polyps.[75] Unfortunately for those patients taking Celebrex, a recent study run by the National Cancer Institute to measure the drug's effectiveness in reducing polyps in people who already had at least one polyp found (at an 800 milligram dose) a 3.4 times increased risk of cardiovascular events.[76] The U.S. Food and Drug Administration now advises doctors to find an alternative pain reliever.[77]

Coffee

The results of a significant study of coffee consumption and lifestyle among 23,912 white Seventh-day Adventists was released in 1984. It showed a positive association between coffee consumption and fatal colon cancers.[78] However a number of more recent studies have found a consistent inverse association between coffee consumption and colon cancer.[79] In those studies the more coffee consumed the less often colon cancer appeared. A review of epidemiological studies, while not advocating coffee as a preventative or treatment, offered several plausible biological explanations—the reductions in cholesterol and bile acids induced by coffee consumption; the antimutagenic properties of selected coffee components; and more frequent bowel movements.[80] Another study published in the *American Journal of Epidemiology* speculated that the individuals at high risk of colorectal cancers may have chosen to avoid drinking coffee, again skewing the results.[81] Health risks associated with coffee are further detailed on pages 98-99.

Garlic

A number of studies provide evidence of the anticarcinogenic effects of the active ingredients in garlic.[82] A critical review of the epidemiologic literature by researchers in the Department of Epidemiology at the University of North Carolina concluded that there is a preventative effect on colorectal cancers from eating cooked or raw garlic.[83]

Meat

A systematic review of 13 studies of the relationship between meat consumption and colorectal cancer was conducted by the University of Cambridge Institute of Public Health.[84] The pooled results showed that as the amount of meat consumed daily increased, so did the risk for cancers of the colon and rectum. For processed meats the picture is even bleaker. The risk grew by nearly 50 percent with a 25-gram daily increase in processed meats.

Fruits and Vegetables

A summary of studies examining the protective effects of fruits and vegetables on cancer risk has been gathered by researchers representing the Unit of Nutrition and Cancer at the International Agency for Research on Cancer. The results support a significant reduction in the risks of colon and rectal cancers in association with the consumption of both fruits and vegetables.[85] Additionally, the results were also clear for cancers of the lungs, esophagus, and stomach. A larger analysis of published studies, systematic reviews, meta-analyses, and large prospective studies by University of Oxford cancer researchers reached the same conclusions about fruits and vegetables.[86] The Oxford study recommends eating 400 grams of fruits and vegetables per day.

Fiber

Confusion surrounds the reasons for the beneficial effects of a fiber-rich diet on the risk of developing colon and rectal cancers. A study of 2,157 people by researchers at the University of Utah found that both soluble and insoluble fiber have a role in preventing rectal cancer.[87] Insoluble fiber speeds the passage of toxins through the system. Soluble fiber creates compounds that stop cancer cell growth while removing tumor-promoting chemicals.[88] A daily serving of five and a half portions of vegetables created a 28 percent drop in rectal cancer risk; three and a half servings of fruit led to a 27 percent drop in rectal cancer risk; just three servings of whole grains generated a 31 percent reduction of risk.[89] The National Cancer Institute uses the following portion sizes in their guidelines: a serving equals a medium piece of fruit, ½ cup of fruit or vegetable, 1 cup of leafy greens, ¼ cup dried fruit, or 6 ounces (¾ cup) of juice.[90] The American Cancer Society recommends increasing the role of fruits and vegetables in the diet, and obtaining our fiber that way instead of through fiber supplements.[91]

Experts are divided about whether the decrease in cancer risk is because of fiber or some other substance in a high-fiber diet. Fiber is thought to dilute carcinogens and decrease their contact with the porous lining of the digestive tract. Fiber binds and inhibits the production of carcinogens. The health-promoting "good" bacteria in the colon flourish in the presence of fiber. The fermentation of fiber in the intestines appears to limit the growth of cancer cells.[92] This is especially true of flaxseed fiber, because it promotes the production of the powerful anti-carcinogen mammalian lignan.[93]

For a while it was thought that fiber reduced the colon polyps that can lead to colon cancer. Some doubt was thrown on this role for fiber by two trials released in 2000.[94] One four-year-long study compared 1,000 people who consumed 33 grams of fiber a day along with six and a half daily servings of fruits and vegetables with 1,000 people who ate their usual diet with about 19 grams of fiber. The two groups had about the same number of polyps. A second three-year-long study compared 700 people who ate 14 grams of wheat bran fiber a day to nearly 600 people who only ate 2 grams of fiber a day and found no significant difference in polyps.

A diagnosis of colon cancer calls for the help of doctors, support groups, and lifestyle adjustments. The role of fiber in producing anticarcinogens, diluting carcinogens, hastening the passage of carcinogens, and helping bacteria to limit the growth of cancer cells makes it an important weapon in the fight against cancer.

Exercise and Weight Maintenance

Nearly 170 epidemiologic studies have been conducted on physical activity as a way to prevent cancer. A report released by researchers Friedenreich and Orenstein of the Division of Epidemiology, Prevention and Screening, of the Alberta Cancer Board classified physical activity as creating a convincing reduction of risk for colon cancers. The research, printed in the *Journal of Nutrition* in November 2002, suggested possible reasons for the benefits of exercise as changes in hormones, growth factors, immune function, and the reduction of fat deposits and obesity.[95]

Being overweight is a risk factor for colon cancer.[96] An American study of over 900,000 adults found that death rates from colon-rectal cancer were 20–84 percent higher in overweight and severely obese men and 10–46 percent higher in overweight and severely obese women compared to normal weight adults.[97] Overweight and obese adults should be screened for colon cancer; early detection and intervention might save their lives. The next step is to reduce the weight.

THE
Weekend Cleanse Plan

Weekend Cleanse Basics

Many elements come together to support the cleansing process. Some of the most crucial elements were covered in previous sections—pure nutritious food and regular elimination. These two factors alone will do wonders to help build a healthy body. To round out the cleansing process, it is valuable to examine the mechanics of how to eat. This involves eating more slowly, chewing well, and appreciating our food. Breathing also comes into play, as the process of breathing cleans out toxins, and awareness of the breath settles the mind.

Having loved ones and mentors is a great treasure, as their support can encourage healing. We must learn to acknowledge and cultivate these relationships.

Exercise saves lives and spreads joy. Our bodies were made for exercise (among other things, of course). Aerobics and resistance training will strengthen the body, encourage nutrients to do their work, and move toxins along their way. There are particular movements that tone the digestive system and help the bowels move.

One of the finest techniques for eliminating toxins is fasting. The weekend fast detailed in this book offers a method to begin using this valuable tool. (Yes, people can skip a day or two of eating and come off a fast in better health.)

All of these components—good nutrition, proper eating, conscious breathing, a supportive network, exercise, and fasting—are brought together in the Weekend Cleanse.

The Weekend Cleanse is a simple two-day program of abstaining from solid foods and getting moderate exercise and plenty of rest. The Weekend Cleanse will release toxins, tune up the digestion, burn off a little weight, teach us important lessons about the body, and move us forward with improved health and digestion. The Weekend Cleanse is a powerful tool but it is not a cure-all. The Weekend Cleanse can rejuvenate the body and prevent the onset of illness. If the Weekend Cleanse becomes a turning point in how and what you eat, if it marks a new readiness to exercise, if the Weekend Cleanse gives you the confidence to make changes in your life and take personal control of your health—that is the measure of success.

Some of the beauty of the Weekend Cleanse is that it can be done without disrupting work schedules. Of course certain weekend activities, such as going out for dinner, may need to be postponed until a better time. Holidays, like Thanksgiving, when family and friends gather to eat in communion, are not good times for a cleanse.

Weekend Cleanse
Drinking Options

Pure Water	or	Pure Water
		Fresh Juice
		Teas
		Kicker Lemonade

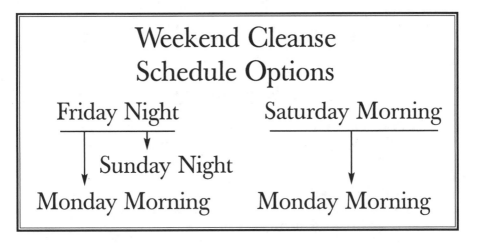

Weekend Cleanse
Schedule Options

Friday Night	Saturday Morning

Sunday Night

Monday Morning · Monday Morning

The Weekend Cleanse should not be done by people with life-threatening diseases such as cancer, AIDs, hepatitis, kidney failure, or tuberculosis. Pregnant or lactating women, infants, and children should not do the Weekend Cleanse. Anyone taking prescription drugs should not undertake the Weekend Cleanse without first consulting with their doctor.

During the Weekend Cleanse eat no fats, oils, starches, or meats. There are two drinking options for the weekend: water only, or liquids such as teas, Kicker Lemonade (page 101), and and/or fresh whole juices. Water is the simplest way to go. Our ancestors faced repeated and extensive periods of no food when only water was available. Our bodies have evolved complex and coordinated mechanisms of survival and healing in the absence of food.[1]

The second decision is to choose when to begin and end the Weekend Cleanse. The best times to start are Friday evening after supper, or Saturday morning after a light breakfast. Resume eating some solid food Sunday night, or wait until Monday morning. I generally recommend waiting until Monday morning, but if you are new to fasting or have other reasons to eat Sunday night, go ahead and come off the fast.

The rest of this section explains pertinent details of the Weekend Cleanse. Take a look at The Weekend Cleanse Day by Day (pages 90-91), which shows where each of these elements comes into play.

The Weekend Cleanse Day by Day

Friday evening

Drink plenty of water
Work out with weights
Eat a light supper
Brush teeth
Long walk before bed
Review goals and motivation
Drink a laxative tea or drink
Get a good night's sleep

Saturday morning

Wake up and drink a glass of room temperature water
Breathing exercises
Shower
Brush teeth
Stretching and elimination exercises
A little coffee, if that is the habit

Saturday (rest of the day)

Drink plenty of water, juice, and/or Kicker Lemonade
Brush teeth
Long walk before bed
Shower
Review goals and motivation
Get a good night's sleep

Sunday morning

Wake up and drink a glass of room temperature water
Breathing exercises
Shower
Brush teeth
Stretching and elimination exercises
A little coffee
Water, juice, and/or Kicker Lemonade

Simple Cleanse

The Weekend Cleanse Day by Day
(continued)

Sunday afternoon/evening

If you have decided beforehand that you are coming off the fast
 tonight, then eat a vegetable salad for supper.
Long walk before bed
Shower
Brush teeth
Review goals and motivation
Get a good night's sleep

Monday

Breathing exercises
Drink a glass of room temperature water
Stretching/elimination exercises
Light breakfast of brown rice or fruit salad
Milk thistle tea or capsules
Resume taking supplements about two hours after breakfast
One or two cups cooked organic brown rice
Enjoy going to work
Small lunch
Small supper
Walk before bed

Tuesday-Thursday

Back to normal—if "normal" is eating a balanced plant-based
 diet with lots of fruit and vegetables. If not—then now is the
 time for permanent change.
Eat sensibly
Drink plenty of water
Exercise
Maintain positive outlook

Thursday or Friday is a time of preparation. Sometimes there is a feeling of tiredness during the cleansing period. If that happens, limit activities that fall into the "must be done" category. Try to rest without concern about tasks to be done. Gather any foods or drinks you'll need for the next three days. If you are cleansing with water only, this will be easy. Also gather foods for coming off the fast. This way they will be available should you decide to change the time of ending the fast. Purchase fresh organic fruits and vegetables. Make sure you have organic brown rice to prepare for coming off the fasting segment of the Weekend Cleanse. Portion out the drinks. Plan on having juices and teas for Saturday and Sunday.

Friday afternoon and evening are good times to practice resistance training or aerobics. It is better to do a good workout on Friday and take it easy over the weekend. It is fine to do some gentle hatha yoga postures throughout the weekend of the cleanse. The increased flexibility you experience may be surprising.

Eat a light meal Friday night. Before you eat give thanks for the food. Give thanks to those who prepared it. Give thanks to those who harvest, to those who sell. Be grateful for this beautiful planet. Pick up the fork. Is there any forgotten blessing for something you are grateful for? Be careful not to overeat tonight. Friday night is a traditional time to kick back and relax after a week of work. Relax your body. Relax your mind. Do not relax your awareness. Eat one helping of a balanced, well-cooked meal, seasoned to taste. Savor each mouthful. When finished, brush your teeth and scrape your tongue. Having clean teeth and tongue will help fend off the urge to eat after supper. Put away the food without picking at the leftovers. Wash the dishes. Clean the kitchen.

After eating each evening, take a walk. It is hard to underestimate the benefits of walking. If walking is not currently a habit, please make it a regular part of your life. Pounds will melt away. Flab will vanish. Lung capacity will increase. The gentle massage given to the bowels by the act of walking stimulates digestion. Nutrients are carried to every part of the body. Cellular waste is passed into the bowels, expelled in the breath, and brought to the surface of the body by sweat.

Walking with friends can be an enjoyable and mutually supportive experience. We can appreciate our surroundings. Our bodies are growing in purity, health, and strength. While walking, begin reviewing your goals and motivation for the cleanse.

Each day of the cleanse take some time to be by yourself. Sitting with a straight, relaxed spine, close your eyes and observe your breath. See how your body is feeling. Pay close attention, especially during a cleansing process. A primary goal is to stay in touch with what your body is telling you. It is okay to stop a cleanse at any point and choose a new direction based on the feedback you receive from your precious body. When we care well for our body, our body will carry us on our journey in this world. If there are questions and the answers are not forthcoming, get the help of a trusted health care professional. Stay in contact with loved ones through any great changes. They can help keep our outlook balanced. Loved ones need to share in our success and joy.

Fasting

Fasting is a well-established technique for removing toxins. When we fast, we purposely abstain from food for a limited time. Fasting has been proven to be effective for a variety of disorders of the stomach and intestines. Fasting improves the healing of diseases of the upper respiratory tract: the nostrils, nasal cavities, and sinuses. Fasting rests the digestive tract while activating stored toxins so they can be flushed from the body.

Fasting puts us in touch with our true sense of hunger. It is important to reconnect with the instinctual urge to eat because we have been socially and personally conditioned to eat types and quantities of food beyond what is needed for our optimum health. There are many types of fasting. More information is known about water fasting than any other natural treatment for healing the body.

In modern times, juice fasting became popularized in Europe. A juice fast can easily transition a person into the fasting state of physiologic rest. Many people in relatively good health can stick with a juice fast for a longer period than a fast on water only. This is because juice provides an easily digestible and absorbable form of food for the cells of the body. Because of the ease of absorption, the digestive system gets a rest while the nutrient levels remain high.

Fasting one day a week for a month or two can strengthen our understanding and physical ability to fast for the two fasting days of the Weekend Cleanse. Fasting is unwise and potentially dangerous for people with a compromised immune system, cancer, diabetes, gout, hypoglycemia, stomach ulcers, or disease of the liver, kidney, or lungs. People in these situations should only fast under direct medical supervision. Pregnant and lactating women should not fast, focusing instead on a healthful diet, exercise, relaxation, and loving relationships. Consult with a health care professional before fasting.

Fasting does not mean to starve the body. Starvation is when the lack of food fuel causes the body to begin burning essential tissue in muscles and organs for energy. The liver, intestines, heart, and kidneys will all lose high percentages of weight when faced with starvation. The shrinking heart begins beating with a slower pulse and with less pressure. Death typically arrives in eight to twelve weeks. Fasting is not starvation.

During a fast the body first utilizes carbohydrates stored in the cells as glycogen. As stored glycogen is depleted, the body begins harvesting fat as the preferred energy source. In this way the protein in muscle tissue is partially spared.

It is possible to lose some muscle tissue even during a short fast. Weakness, nausea, headaches, and depression can also develop during a fast, because toxins that had been stored in fat are being released. Additional stress can be placed on the kidneys by ketones, by-products of fat metabolism. It is important to drink plenty of pure water during a fast to help flush the kidneys. The breakdown of muscle tissue will release ammonia and nitrogen into the blood. Extended fasts, in extreme situations, can lead to disturbances of the heart's rhythm and ultimately death.

The safest fast is a short fast like the Weekend Cleanse, which lasts one or two days. Consult with a health care professional if there is any reason to think your health might preclude a fast. Even a healthy person wishing to fast more than two to three days should be medically supervised.

Simple Cleanse

During a fast, persistent organic pollutants and other toxins that have been stored in the fatty tissues can be released. Concentrations of toxins passing into the urine and stool increase during a fast. The release of toxins can generate symptoms such as headaches, nausea, fatigue, sweating, sore throat, runny nose, achy joints, palpitations, and dizziness. Although these may be side effects of fasting, they can also be caused by other serious medical problems. For this reason it is important to have a health care professional assisting anyone on a fast.

On one level the presentation of symptoms is a good sign that the body is processing toxins. However this is also a signal to slow down the cleanse. Drink some juice. If you still don't feel well after an hour or two, eat half a cup of cooked brown rice. If the symptoms pass, continue the fast. If the symptoms persist, gradually come off the fast by eating another half cup of brown rice or half a banana. Wait another hour or two and have more brown rice or banana.

Sleep

Get a good night's sleep. Sleep is critical to health. This is a time for the body to work at breaking down and eliminating wastes without serving the impulsive desires of the waking mind. If you experience fatigue during the days of the Weekend Cleanse, take a nap. No problem.

Teeth

Brush your teeth each morning of the Weekend Cleanse. Some people may wonder why it is important to brush our teeth in the morning, especially after having brushed them the evening before and consuming no food since then. The yellowish residue that builds up on the tongue and teeth as we sleep must be dealt with. Brush it off. A valuable tool for dental care is a specialized toothbrush with narrow, cone-shaped bristles that get into the spaces between the teeth and along the gum. If there is room between the teeth for the bristles of this type of toothbrush, then get in there and scrub those surfaces. Bacteria that live in the mouth can enter the bloodstream and infect the valves and inner lining of the heart, a condition known as bacterial endocarditis.[2] There are several commercially produced scrapers to clean the surface of the tongue. First-time users who clean the tongue are in for both a shock at the residue they'll remove and a pleasant surprise at the feeling of a clean tongue. A clean mouth is a healthy mouth.

Bathing

The evening shower is a healthful practice with blessings ranging from the tactile sensations of water and temperature to the shedding of dirt, bacteria, old skin, and the toxins brought to the surface from organs and tissues deep in the body. Grandma said, "Cleanliness is next to godliness," the reason being that a clean body promotes the forces of healing.

The skin is considered by naturopaths to be the largest of our eliminative organs; they believe sweating is a powerful way to expel accumulated toxins.[3] We each have two kinds of sweat glands—eccrine and apocrine. Together there are four or five million of these tiny glands distributed over our body. About three million of these glands are eccrine glands that secrete an odorless, clear fluid that cools the body by evaporating. The main function of sweat is to regulate body temperature. A bead of sweat the size of a pea can cool nearly one liter of blood one degree Fahrenheit.[4] Even modest increases in the temperature of the human brain can be dangerous or fatal. A theory advanced by brain researcher Dean Falk suggests the human brain can grow no larger than the cooling system attached to it.[5] Apocrine sweat glands start working at puberty and open into hair follicles located in limited areas—such as the armpits and genital regions. In nonhuman mammals the apocrine sweat releases pheromones that signal mating behavior. This could be the case in humans also, but the connection may be obscured by social behavior and has not been subjected to scientific verification. Apocrine glands produce a thick, odorless fluid, rich in organic substances, that is decomposed on the surface of the skin by bacteria that produce strong odors. Sweat is about 99 percent water; the remaining 1 percent is salt, fat molecules, vitamin C, lactic acid, nickel, urea, and manufactured drugs and their by-products. Talk to your health care practitioner if you notice a change in body odor, because it may signal a medical condition. A fruity smell may be a sign of diabetes. The smell of ammonia may indicate liver or kidney disease. Wash your body. Keep your pores healthy and functioning properly. Sweat. It will save a host of problems.

Supplements and Medications

During the Weekend Cleanse most common supplements can be skipped without ill effect. The best way to get vitamins and minerals is in their original package—fruits, vegetables, and whole grains. If you are concerned about missing vital minerals or vitamins, juice the vegetables or fruits that naturally contain those nutrients. People on medications should consult with their health care professional before trying the Weekend Cleanse.

Light Laxatives

My favorite laxative is psyllium seed husks. In our digestive tract, psyllium has attributes of both soluble and insoluble fiber. Psyllium husks are the most successful fiber for catching and passing toxins and cholesterol. Psyllium husks expand in water 10–15 times their weight to form a soft bulk that moves easily through the intestines.[6] Mix a level tablespoon of psyllium husks in an 8–12-ounce glass of water. Stir with vigor and drink it before the husks settle. The drink has a pleasant nutty flavor. Continue to drink plenty of water until the bowels move. John Harvey Kellogg learned about psyllium during a visit to Sicily, and introduced it to the United States at the Battle Creek Sanitarium.[7]

Laxative teas are a soothing way to begin a cleanse. There are a number of laxative tea mixes on the market. I prefer teas made from only one herb so I can tell what that ingredient does to my body. Others may prefer a mix, either commercially available or a blend of their own choosing.

Tea

There are a number of pleasant, unsweetened teas you can sip during the two days of the Weekend Cleanse. In the evening sip a cup of lemon balm tea. Lemon balm is a sedative. Although the FDA recognizes lemon balm as safe, some herbalists suggest not operating motorized vehicles after drinking lemon balm tea. Not only is lemon balm itself a sedative, there is some evidence that it may increase the sedative effects of other drugs.[8]

Milk thistle is a bitter tea that will rejuvenate the liver. Milk thistle combines an increased secretion and flow of bile with antioxidant properties and support for ribonucleic acid (RNA), working with DNA to bring about protein synthesis. The primary active ingredient in milk thistle seed is silymarin. Silymarin protects liver cells as they process toxins; it also helps to rebuild damaged liver tissue.[9]

Peppermint tea is a pleasant, calming tea that will reduce nausea and settle the fasting stomach. Taken while not fasting, it aids in digestion and the reduction of flatulence.

Slippery elm bark makes a soothing tea that will reduce inflammation in the colon.[10] Teas including slippery elm bark are available at most health food stores.

Coffee

Coffee can stimulate the bowels to move. If you are normally a coffee drinker, there is little harm in drinking a small amount of coffee in the morning. Not only does coffee get the bowels moving, it may be just the pick-me-up you need to go forth into the world. There are health promoters who argue vociferously against drinking coffee for several reasons. The most compelling arguments against coffee drinking concern its ability to raise blood pressure and increase the risk of urinary tract cancer.[11]

Research conducted by Michael J. Klag, MD, director of the Division of General Internal Medicine at Johns Hopkins, involving 1,000 men found that coffee drinkers had a 28 percent incidence of hypertension compared to a 19 percent incidence of hypertension within a control group of men who did not drink coffee. The coffee drinkers were also more likely to smoke cigarettes and drink alcohol than the men who avoided coffee, which may have skewed the results.[12] Noting other studies showing that avoiding caffeine can lower blood pressure, Dr. Klag recommends that people with high blood pressure reduce their coffee consumption. A meta-analysis using statistical methods to combine the results of 23 studies found "very little excess risk of coronary heart disease among habitual coffee drinkers," but there was a possibility of "increased risk of heart disease among a subgroup of people who acutely increased their coffee intake."[13]

There is good reason to think there is a connection between urinary tract cancer and coffee, so caution is encouraged. In 1985 the *Journal of the American Dietary Association* published a review of 18 years of research on the carcinogenic effects of both caffeine and coffee that concluded "no causal relationship has been established between coffee intake and lower urinary tract cancer."[14] However more recently (2001) a systematic review and meta-analysis of 37 studies concluded that coffee consumption increased the risk of urinary tract cancer by approximately 20 percent.[15]

Whatever you decide about using coffee, decide prior to your fast. For most heavy consumers of caffeine, the Weekend Cleanse may not be the best time to quit drinking coffee, although some may view this as an opportunity to shed a habit they have outgrown.

Water

For a steady fast it is best to drink only water during the cleanse. Drink 8–10 glasses of water a day. Adequate hydration will help flush out disease-provoking toxins. The kidneys rarely pause in their efforts to wash fluid waste from the body, even during the Weekend Cleanse. On a normal day the urinary system will filter 500 gallons of blood. The urine will pass environmental toxins converted by the liver and "cellular wastes" such as urea and ammonia produced during protein metabolism. The kidneys work hard and need water to function properly.

Juice

Juice can be used for several purposes during the Weekend Cleanse. If you are fasting on water you might want to switch to juice toward the end of the cleanse as a way to ease back into solid food, or you may feel you need the nutrients supplied by juice to carry on your activities during the Weekend Cleanse.

To accelerate the cleanse, drink a little organic fruit juice. Apple is a good choice. Organic cherry juice is my personal favorite for flushing out any remaining wads of mucus. It is nice to finish up on Sunday evening by drinking up to a quart of organic juice. That will clean out the majority of the intestinal residue that has accumulated over the weekend.

Freshly juiced apples are a rich source of the multipurpose health builder fruit pectin. Fruit pectin cleanses the intestinal tract while lowering cholesterol and blood glucose. Although pectin is found in the highest concentrations in apples, it is also abundant in citrus fruits and is found to some extent in all fruits and vegetables. Beneficial intestinal flora thrives on pectin, helping to keep harmful bacteria and yeasts in check while synthesizing B vitamins. Pectin allows the helpful intestinal bacteria to produce short-chain fatty acids that act as a nutrient to the lining of the intestinal tract, protecting against cancer and upholding the integrity of the colon. Additionally pectin helps the body to pass heavy metals such as beryllium, manganese, mercury, and especially lead.[16]

Juice is the way to get concentrated nutrition in an easily assimilated form. Even if a person is suffering from weak digestion, juice will offer up 99 percent of its food value.[17] Try carrot juice. A pound of organic carrots will make a large glass of delicious carrot juice. We would have real trouble eating that many carrots but no trouble drinking all the enzymes, minerals, water-soluble vitamins, and trace elements extracted from that pound of carrots.[18] During the week juices provide the supplemental vitamins and minerals our bodies crave. During the Weekend Cleanse they are essential foods.

Kicker Lemonade

There are a number of ways to prepare lemonade for a cleanse. Choose large, heavy lemons with thin skin and a bright yellow color. Organic lemons are best. Wash the lemons thoroughly before cutting them open for juicing. Start with the juice of about half a lemon in an 8-ounce glass of water. Adjust the strength to taste, adding as much lemon juice as seems appropriate. Do not drink so much that your belly hurts. Pain in the stomach area is an indication to back off the fast.

Sweeten the lemon water to taste with one to three tablespoons of a complex natural sweetener. Do not use white sugar. Honey is absorbed quickly into the system and may be used in the Weekend Cleanse for short bursts of energy. People with diabetes should not use sugar or honey and should further consult with their heath care practitioners about all of the ingredients and methods used in a cleanse before beginning. Pure maple syrup is an excellent sweetener, as are agave syrup, sorghum syrup, and brown rice syrup.

To spice the lemonade with a little "heat," add some mucus-dissolving cayenne. A few shakes will do it. A glass of this invigorating drink will reveal how it gets the name Kicker Lemonade.

Coming Off the Weekend Cleanse

How to Eat

How food is eaten can be as important as what is eaten. Poor digestion can result from bad eating habits. Some of these habits may go on for years before the cumulative effects make themselves known. Digestion will improve if our awareness of what we eat and the feelings we experience as we eat translate into improved eating habits.

A good method for slowing down and maintaining conscious awareness while we eat is the act of saying grace at the beginning of a meal. Religious cultures throughout the human family employ this technique, but it is not necessary to practice a religion to take a quiet moment before eating to appreciate the food. Although fostering an attitude of gratitude is not the only benefit of prayer or meditation before eating, it is primary and nearly universal.

It is important to relax while eating. Eating in a hurry usually means inadequate chewing, swallowing more air, and experiencing heartburn, belching, bloating, and gas. Who needs it? Relax. Give food a good chew. Appreciate its taste. Chew it well and savor the subtle flavors. Do not stress out. Especially do not stress about digestion. Stress interferes with the normal activity of the intestines, causing a variety of "sick" stomach problems including bloating and constipation or diarrhea.

Eat tasty food of high quality. Don't go for bulk. Overeating is a common bad habit. Our appetites are greater than our needs. Mahatma Gandhi used to say, "True happiness is impossible without true health, and true health is impossible without a rigid control of the palate."[19] Or, as Grandma would admonish me, "Don't let your eyes be bigger than your stomach." Overeating is common everywhere in the world that people can afford to eat whatever they want. The body is capable of producing only a limited volume of digestive fluids at any given time. Eating large amounts of food at one sitting puts a heavy burden on the digestive system. Some food is not even digested or utilized by the body. What a waste of food, money, and time, not to mention the physical discomfort and potential weight gain. Moderate portions are more easily digested. The dietary genius Steve Meyerowitz, a.k.a. "Sproutman," writes, "Overconsumption is the number one cause of indigestion." And worse: "Man can survive on one-third of his daily food intake. The other two-thirds goes to the benefit of the health insurance and medical care industries."[20]

The timing of food consumption is often regulated by the schedule of others rather the actual needs of our bodies. Eating on a regular schedule of our own choosing and regularly eating the same or similar foods aids digestion. An orderly entry ensures an orderly passage. People in the developed world who eat at regular intervals tend to eat more nutritious foods than those who eat at irregular intervals.[21] Skipping meals can increase the appetite and lead to overeating.

Potential Side Effects of the Weekend Cleanse

As the body begins releasing and processing toxins, you may experience various "symptoms." You may get headaches, nausea, dizziness, mood swings, and/or achy muscles. Some of this is to be expected when toxins are flushed from their hidden lairs. If these side effects are disturbing, gently come off the cleanse by eating half a banana or a half cup of cooked brown rice. Then wait an hour or so and eat a little more. The cleanse is intended to improve our health, but we are all unique and need to judge the efficacy of these techniques for ourselves and adjust them accordingly.

Some people like the effects of the Weekend Cleanse so much that they want to continue it for longer periods of time. Before experimenting further, consult your health care professional.

Maintaining

The most important ways to maintain the positive effects of the Weekend Cleanse are to eat right, exercise, sleep, and cleanse regularly. Try doing the Weekend Cleanse once every month or so, up to five times a year. It is also healthful to fast one day a week. I find it most convenient to fast the same day each week. Any day is good if you can maintain your regular schedule or if you are able to get some downtime.

Other Aspects of Cleansing

Breath of Life

We are born breathing, but we don't often think about it. Mostly our breath takes care of itself. We simply breathe and stay alive. It is usually so effortless that it is easy to take our breath for granted.

Oxygen is our most important nutrient, even though we worry more about food. Are we eating too much or too little? Are we eating the right amounts of the right foods? Some folks wonder where their next meal will come from. But people who are in good health can go for weeks without food. People can even live without water for days. But the breath? Six minutes without air and the brain begins to die. Life hinges on our next breath.

The role of the breath in purifying and cleansing the physical body is critical in three important ways. The breath is an oxygen delivery system, a waste transport system, and a primary mover of the lymphatic system. (See Lymph, page 52.)

The breath purifies the blood by accepting toxins through the porous walls of the alveoli—tender bags that blossom like flowers in the lungs. Spiraling winds of oxygenated air enter our nostrils as the diaphragm drops and the lungs expand. Oxygen is a catalyst for change and renewal. Oxygen is carried by a wild flood of red blood cells to each corner of the fantastically intricate coordinated whole of our body.

The lungs expel more than just carbon dioxide. They also outgas water vapor, hydrogen, methane, and small amounts of toxins that are released by capillaries deep in the alveoli of the lungs.

A pioneering study on the role of the breath in stimulating and cleansing the lymph was conducted by Jack Shields, MD, a lymphologist at the Department of Medicine and Hematology, Santa Barbara Medical Foundation Clinic, California.[22] Using cameras to observe the interface between the diaphragm and the lymphatic system, he observed lymphatic movement proportional to the volume of air inspired with each breath. Deep diaphragmatic breathing created a vacuum effect that sucked the lymph along its course.

When breathing is rapid and irregular, the mind is disturbed and thinking is erratic. Long, slow, deep breathing is easier on the nervous system. With regular breathing the metabolism stabilizes and digestion comes more easily. Peaceful, orderly breathing settles the mind. The body follows the mind. Our thoughts rise and fall with the breath. In rhythm with the breath think: "May all those in pain be healed. May all beings be happy. May all beings be free." When thoughts arise, look at them but do not dwell on them. Do not dwell on positive thoughts. Do not dwell on negative thoughts. They will all pass. The ancient Chinese sage Chuang Tzu teaches: "Emptiness is the fasting of the mind."[23]

Sinus Cleansing

The mucus and hairs in the nasal passages trap toxic particles and keep them from getting into the lungs. To keep the sinuses clean and our breath free and unobstructed, it is wise to gently clean the nasal passages with a little salt water. Yoga practitioners and ayurvedic healers have done this since ancient times. Salt water is healing. The technique of cleaning the nasal passages is to use water with about the same salt content of tears to flush out pollutants, pollens, bacteria, and other particles. To get the right concentration of salt that works best for you may take a little experimentation, but the reward is well worth the effort. Use sea salt and begin with about ¼ rounded teaspoon of salt dissolved in eight ounces of water. After trying that amount a few times, gradually increase the salt to about ½ rounded teaspoon per eight ounces of water. Always use lukewarm water. This is much more soothing than cold water. Hot water will injure the mucous membranes.

There are two main ways of introducing the salt water into the nasal passages: the first is what I call the "at hand method," snorting from the cupped palm; the other is pouring the solution from a neti pot. The advantage of using the cupped palm is that it is free and you always have it with you. The disadvantages are that some people find the act of snorting irritating to the mucous membranes, and it tends to be a little messy. Salt water will likely enter the mouth and will need to be spit out. The neti pot is usually a small cup or bowl-shaped container with a cone-shaped spout, similar to a tiny teapot. The neti pot allows a more controlled and gentle experience. It is possible to breathe calmly through the mouth while using the neti pot. With a little practice the water will flow into one nostril and out the other. Both methods are easy.

To use the "at hand method," pour a little of the lukewarm salt water into the cupped palm of your hand. Gently pressing one nostril closed with your thumb or finger, snort the salt water up through the other nostril. Let the salt water find its way from the first nasal passage into the other nasal passage or the mouth and allow it to run out. Blow gently and clean. Then do the same with the other nostril. Any leftover salt water can be used after brushing to gargle and rinse the mouth.

To use the neti pot method, just tilt your head to one side and insert the spout into the highest nostril. Before allowing any salt water to flow through the spout, be sure there is a seal between the spout and the inside rim of the nostril. (You may need to shop around a little to find the right width spout for your nostrils.) Lift the bowl of the neti pot so the water flows into one nostril and out the other. If the solution drains into the mouth, just spit it out and gargle when done. To avoid getting any in the mouth, increase the tilt of your head. Rinse the other nostril the same way. Blow gently and clean.

Bellows Breath

Here is an exercise to be done at least two hours after eating: To stimulate deep diaphragmatic breathing, relax the abdomen. Let the diaphragm drop down, then inhale and expand the chest. To exhale, first deflate the chest, then pull the diaphragm up and in. The basic motion of the diaphragm is to drop down to expand the lungs and to contract upward to expel the air.

There is an even more powerful breath for cleaning and releasing toxins from the lungs, blood vessels, and cells—the deep and rapid diaphragmatic breathing called the Bellows Breath.

The focus of the Bellows Breath is on the navel point. This is a fairly rapid breathing rhythm, up to two breaths per second with no pause between the inhalation and exhalation. Begin learning and practicing very slowly. A quicker pace can come later. Relax the body and sit with a straight spine. The head, neck, and trunk should be in line. Keep the chest area moderately relaxed throughout the exercise. Begin the breath by pulling in the navel and abdomen towards the spine, pushing the air out of the lungs. Without pausing, inhale by gently thrusting the navel forward while using the abdominal muscles to bring the diaphragm down. This will draw fresh air into the lungs. Balance the length of time of the inhalation with the exhalation, making them equal.

This is a wonderful cleansing breath if done correctly. Experiencing light-headedness is a signal to stop. We do not want to pass out and become injured falling! If there is a dizzy or "heady" feeling, the Bellows Breath is being done incorrectly. The most common error is breathing from the upper part of the lungs. That produces hyperventilation and is not the Bellows Breath. The problem with hyperventilation is that it decreases carbon dioxide in the arteries. The reduction of arterial carbon dioxide constricts the small arteries and arterioles that feed the brain and spinal cord. If dizziness occurs, gently lie on your back and breathe abdominally with your hands or a light weight on your abdomen. It is possible to gradually work up to a few minutes of the Bellows Breath. This energizes the body, moves lymph, clears toxins, and aids digestion. Try it.

Mild aerobic exercise will stimulate breathing and cleanse the lungs. Singing will work wonders for the lungs. We should sing loudly every day, without caring who hears. Life is sweet.

A Word About Tobacco Use

Tobacco is nasty and addictive. It negatively affects every part of the digestive system. No matter how a person uses it (smoked or chewed) or lets it use them, tobacco is a major cause of cancer of the mouth, larynx, pharynx, esophagus, stomach, and pancreas. Additionally, each method of ingesting tobacco has its own special digestive cancer areas. Smoking increases the risk of cancer to the kidneys and bladder. Spit tobacco is a risk factor for prostate cancer.

Cancer is not the only way tobacco attacks the digestive system. Smoking contributes to heartburn, peptic ulcers, and increases the risk of Crohn's disease and gallstones. Tobacco smoke also taxes the liver, working it overtime to remove toxins such as benzopyrene, polycyclic aromatic hydrocarbons, cyanide, acetaldehyde, and tars.[24] The reduced ability of the liver to process toxins, drugs, and alcohol leaves the smoker exposed to dozens of diseases. Nicotine from smoking or chewing tobacco increases the production of stomach acid and decreases production of sodium bicarbonate. Air swallowed while smoking causes bloating and belching. But if someone is hooked on tobacco, burping noxious gas is among the least of their digestive problems.

The good news is that smokers can quit. Millions of people have done it. I quit. Twice, actually. The last time was over 30 years ago. The sense of mental liberation and the energy of expanded lungs and stamina make the struggle worth it.

EXERCISE

Please don't groan. This is where we examine the benefits of exercise. Exercise is good for us. It feels good. We will feel better, look better, and have healthier bowels if we exercise regularly. Exercise works in a variety of ways to reduce stress and tone the digestive system. The main types of exercise recommended for the bowels are aerobic, resistance, and hatha yoga. While exploring these and other exercises we can feel free to gently experiment and develop variations that are best suited to our personal needs. Before beginning any exercise regimen, including weight lifting, resistance training, aerobics, and yoga, consult with your physician or health care provider.

The critical ingredients of aerobic exercise are sustained physical activity that stimulates breathing and increases the heart rate. The activity of the intestinal muscles will be energized, helping to move chyme through the intestines. Exercise can defeat constipation by diverting our thoughts from working cares or household worries, thus conferring the sense of relaxation that facilitates a bowel movement.[1] Aerobic exercise will also improve the heart and lungs, strengthen the immune system, build stamina, and stimulate weight loss.

One of the finest mildly aerobic exercises is simple walking. Walking works wonders, is inexpensive, and convenient. Beginning walkers ought to try 20 minutes a day for a month. They will be happy to see the digestion improving and the pounds melting.

Even eating can pass as exercise if we are eating fiber. Intestinal musculature is improved by working with fibrous dietary bulk. Indigestible material gives the intestinal muscles something to "work against."

Exercising the trunk, especially the abdominal wall and back, helps keep the intestine in its proper place and provides structures with good tone for the intestine to work against. Most traditional cultures have dance movements that exercise the trunk, back, and abdominal muscles.[2]

Having weights or other resistance to work against develops muscles. Our muscles want to work. Lift some weights without overdoing it. See how you feel the next day. Pay attention to how your muscles feel after working out with weights. After a day of rest, work them again. Repeat this cycle and gain strength and vibrancy. It is not only by adding weight that muscles are strengthened. Increasing the repetitions builds muscle tissue. As you add more repetitions, be sure to maintain good form. Strength will increase. Digestion will improve. Fat will vanish. Risk of diabetes, heart disease, and osteoporosis will decrease. Confidence will build.

Toilet Exercises

There are a number of exercises that are best done while sitting on the toilet. The purpose of toilet exercises is twofold. The primary goal is to ease constipation and create comfortable elimination. The secondary aim is to tone and strengthen the abdominal region. The standing exercises and leg lifts have the same goals only reversed. Those exercises are primarily to tone and strengthen the entire abdominal region. In all of the exercises the bowels will be stimulated. If there is an urge to move the bowels, honor that feeling when it occurs.

The general protocol for the toilet exercise is to move the bowels by following the natural flow of the intestines. The natural flow can be traced with your hands. Begin by tracing the course of the ascending colon. First touch the lower right side of your front abdominal region near the front tip of the pelvic girdle. Deeper into the body is where the small intestine enters the large intestine. Move your hands up to just below the lower tip of the rib cage. That area is the ascending colon. The next portion of the large intestine is the transverse colon. Trace it from just below the right rib cage by moving your hands horizontally toward just below the left rib cage. As you move through this area you may feel the diaphragm moving with each breath. The transverse colon is nestled just below the diaphragm. The transverse colon arches slightly inward just below the left rib cage. The intestine begins to turn and angle down from this point. This part of the large intestine is called the descending colon. You can trace it by moving your hands down along the left side of the abdominal cavity. Out of the reach of the fingertips, the sigmoid colon twists back toward the anus for the elimination of stool.

Relax and enjoy these exercises. While sitting on the toilet, keep your feet flat on the floor or slightly raised on a low stool. It may take a little experimentation to find the best foot position. Change and adapt the exercises in this section as necessary.

Side Stretch

This stretch can be done while standing with your feet in line directly under your hips, or while sitting on the toilet with your feet flat on the floor. Place one hand on your hip, if standing, or on your thigh, if sitting. Inhale and arch the other arm straight up, pressing the arm against your ear. Exhale and stretch. Inhale while reversing arms.

Sitting Left Side Stretch

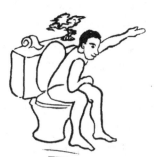

Sitting Side Stretch

Sit erect on the toilet, both of your hands resting on your lap, elbows close to your sides. Inhale as you swing your straightened left arm in an arch above your head. The arm should rest lightly along your ear. Exhale while gently bending and stretching to the right, leading with your raised left hand. The right side of your abdominal region should be pressed between your right forearm and the weight of your body leaning over your forearm. This will put pressure on your ascending colon. Inhale as you come back to sitting erect.

Repeat the Sitting Left Side Stretch two or three more times.

Abdominal Squeeze One

Sit straight and erect with your feet about shoulder width apart or slightly wider. Breathe fully and gently through your nose. Feel supported by your feet and the seat. Relax your shoulders and arms, and rest your hands on your lap.

Inhale as you lift your arms into a bowl shape with the fingertips of each hand lightly touching in front of your chest. Your arms should be in a rounded position, as if gently hugging a tree. Continue inhaling while lifting your arms above your head. Exhale with a slow and controlled breath, leaning forward, pressing the abdominal region against your thighs. Move your hands to your knees to steady the body as you inhale and return to sitting erect with your hands resting on your lap.

Repeat this movement two more times.

Abdominal Squeeze Two

Sit straight and erect with your feet about shoulder width apart or slightly wider. Breathe fully and gently through your nose. Feel supported by your feet and the seat. Relax your shoulders and arms, and rest your lightly clenched fists on your thighs.

Inhale. Exhale with a slow and controlled breath, leaning forward, pressing your abdominal region against the closed fists still resting on your thighs. Rock from side to side to massage the intestinal region. Inhale while sitting back up.

Repeat this movement two or three more times.

Sitting Right Side Stretch

Sit erect on the toilet, both of your hands resting on your lap, elbows close to your sides. Inhale and lift your straightened right arm in an arch over your head. The arm should rest lightly along your ear. Exhale while gently bending and stretching to the left, leading with your raised right hand. The left side of your abdominal region should be pressed between your left forearm and the weight of your body leaning over your forearm. This will put stimulating pressure on your descending colon. Inhale as you come back to sitting erect.

Repeat the Sitting Right Side Stretch two or three more times.

Standing Exercises

Standing Side Stretch

Standing Side Stretch

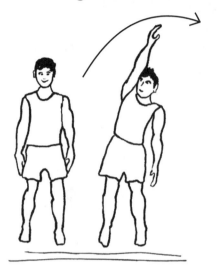

Inhale and lift your right arm straight above your head. The arm should rest lightly along your ear. Exhale while gently bending and stretching to the left, leading with your raised right hand. Inhale as you come back to the upright position. Exhale as you lower your right arm and raise your left arm. Inhale and repeat the movement, this time stretching to the right.

Repeat the Standing Side Stretch two more times.

Lifting Wings

Stand straight and tall, with your feet about shoulder width apart. Breathe fully and gently. Let your feet ground into the floor. From the abdomen up, let your body rise, as though it were suspended by a thread from the crown of your head to the sky. Exhale and relax your shoulders and arms.

Slowly inhale, lifting your arms out from your sides like great wings. Raise your arms together and touch your fingertips overhead. Exhale with a slow and controlled breath, as you lower your arms down to your sides.

Repeat this movement two more times.

Back Arch

Stand with your arms relaxed at your sides. Inhale and raise your arms in unison in front of your body and overhead. Put your palms together. Do not complete the inhalation with your arms above your head. Instead, while still inhaling, gently stretch your arms back, softly arching your back into a gentle curve. Do not push yourself.

Continue to inhale as you straighten your torso, raising your arms, palms together above your head. Hold your arms parallel, lightly pressing against the ears. Keep your feet parallel and your knees straight. Exhale as you lower your arms to your sides. Breathe deeply while relaxing.

Repeat the Back Arch two more times.

For additional stretching, instead of pausing after you complete the Back Arch, inhale, then exhale as you gently bend forward and reach toward your toes. Inhale as you return to an upright position.

Standing Head to Knees

Stand straight and tall, with your feet about shoulder width apart. Breathe fully and gently. Let your feet ground into the floor. From the abdomen up, let your body rise, as though it were suspended by a thread from the crown of your head to the sky. Relax your shoulders and arms.

Slowly inhale, lifting your arms like great wings. Raise your arms above your head, bringing your palms together.

Keeping your palms joined and your extended arms lightly touching your ears, exhale and slowly bend forward, moving your fingertips toward your feet. Bend your knees slightly. There should be no discomfort while performing this movement. Let your hands rest wherever they comfortably reach—along your legs or on the floor. Use your hands and arms to help support

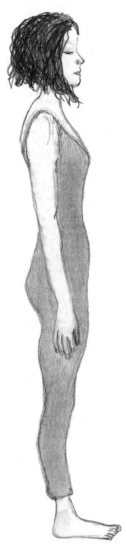

your body. Straighten your legs. Breathe easily in this position. Raise your hips and stretch them toward the sky. Relax your forehead toward your knees.

Inhale, bend your knees slightly, and slowly straighten your back, bringing your arms to a relaxed position hanging alongside your body. Exhale. Breathe evenly.

Inhale and raise your arms like great wings above your head. Exhale and lower them back down.

Repeat the full movement one more time.

Stand relaxed and allow the breath to return to normal.

**Stand Straight
and Tall**

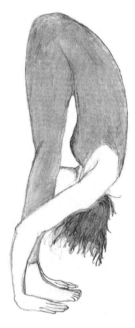

**Forehead Toward
the Knees**

Floor Exercises

To tone and strengthen the abdominal and lumbar (back) muscles, try these leg lifts. Be sure to keep your neck and shoulders relaxed, your legs straight, and your back firmly pressed against the floor while doing the Leg Lift Series. No one should strain to do the exercises. Stay within your body's comfort range.

Rock Pose

Among the premier techniques for reducing stress and toning the bowels are those that have grown out of the ancient teachings of hatha yoga. Perfect digestion does not mean everything can be digested. The only claim that approaches that is a posture called the Rock Pose, supposedly because a person sitting in the Rock Pose can digest even rocks. A Sikh named Guru Bhachan Singh taught me some of the finer points of the Rock Pose. I cannot testify about digesting rocks, but I have gotten hours of service from the pose–time I spent burping and passing gas. You can come into the Rock Pose and test its value for yourself.

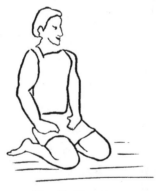

Rock Pose

On a comfortable rug or mat, sit on your knees and feet with your heels pressed lightly into the cheeks of your buttocks. Keep your shoulders raised with a natural curvature in your back. Rest your hands on the tops of your thighs. Breathe evenly through your nose. That's it. Hold the pose as long as seems comfortable. If the feet "fall asleep" or the legs cramp gently come out of the Rock Pose. Do not try the Rock Pose if there are any problems with your knees.

Corpse Pose

The starting and finishing positions for the Leg Lift Series and the Sitting Forward Bend Series are identical. Lie quietly on your back with your legs extended and about shoulder width apart. Your arms should be extended at about a 45-degree angle, your palms relaxed and facing upward. This is the Corpse Pose. Return to it between leg lifts. It is fine to use a couple blankets— one to lie on and another blanket as a cover.

Single Leg Lifts

Lying in the Corpse Pose, bring your arms in close to your sides and bring your heels together. Keep your lower back flattened against the floor. Lift one leg at a time, straight up and straight down, inhaling as you raise the leg and exhaling as you lower it. Coordinate the movement of the leg and the breath. Lowering the leg should take about the same length of time as raising the leg. Begin by raising each leg three times. As your strength increases, repetitions can increase. People with lower back problems, high blood pressure, hiatal hernia, inguinal hernia, stomach ulcers, or duodenal ulcers should not do this exercise.

Double Leg Lifts

This requires more strength than the Single Leg Lifts.

Lying in the Corpse Pose, bring your arms in close to your sides and bring your heels together. Keep your lower back flattened against the floor. Lift both legs at the same time, keeping your knees straight. Use your breath to control the movement. Inhale as you raise your legs and exhale as you lower them. It is all right to take a brief pause at the end of each lift and descent.

Lower your legs in unison, slowly and with control. Smoothly move through a series of three Double Leg Lifts. As your strength increases, repetitions can increase. People with lower back problems, high blood pressure, hiatal hernia, inguinal hernia, stomach ulcers, or duodenal ulcers should not do this exercise.

Crunches

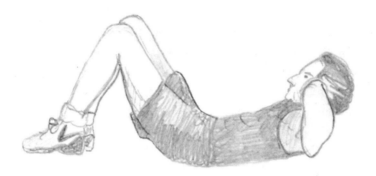

This is a relatively safe exercise that will tone and strengthen the muscles of your abdominal region. Strength and toning will help keep those coils of intestines in place and give you a strong foundation for any other physical activity.

Lie on your back and bend your knees to a comfortable 45-degree angle, drawing your feet in toward your hips. The soles of your feet should be flat on the floor. Interlock your fingers behind your head. Do not force your head forward against the natural inclination of your neck. Using your abdominal muscles, raise your upper body up so that your shoulders lift off the floor. Exhale while your shoulders raise and inhale as your back returns to the floor. Lower yourself down gently. Repeat the exercise as many times as seems appropriate. People with lower back problems, high blood pressure, hiatal hernia, inguinal hernia, stomach ulcers, or duodenal ulcers should not do this exercise.

Laid-back Bicycle

Possibly the best abdominal exercise is the Laid-back Bicycle. Do not be fooled by the name "laid-back," as this exercise can be challenging. Lie on a comfortable surface such as a rug, blanket, or yoga mat. Carefully press your lower back to the floor. Place your hands, palms up, beside your head, touching your fingertips behind your ears. Do not force your head forward against the natural inclination of your neck. Bring your feet off the floor by bending your knees to a 45-degree angle. Slowly and methodically move the legs in a pedaling motion. Alternately touching each elbow to the opposite knee will lift and strengthen the "belly muscles"—rectus abdominus and the obliques. People with lower back problems, high blood pressure, hiatal hernia, inguinal hernia, stomach ulcers, or duodenal ulcers should not do this exercise.

Sitting Forward Bend Series

The Sitting Forward Bend Series is done while sitting on the floor. These movements will tone the internal organs, invigorate the nervous system, and keep the spine supple.

Sitting Head to Knee

Sitting Head to Knee is a posture that requires relaxing into position. Do not force this position. Sit upright on the floor with your legs extended straight out in front. Keep the natural curve in the lower part of your back. Inhale while raising both arms parallel and above your head. Exhale while leaning forward, bending from the hips. Keep your legs straight but do not lock your knees, and reach as far as is comfortable down your legs, even to your feet or beyond. Gently hold your lower legs or toes and draw your chest as close to the tops of your thighs as possible while keeping your spine as straight as possible. Relax your neck and shoulders. Do not force your head down. Hold for 30 seconds. Inhale, keeping the stretch in your back and torso, while raising your torso back into the upright seated position.

Repeat the Sitting Head to Knee Pose two or three more times.

People with knee problems, lower back problems, high blood pressure, hiatal hernia, inguinal hernia, stomach ulcers, or duodenal ulcers should not do this exercise.

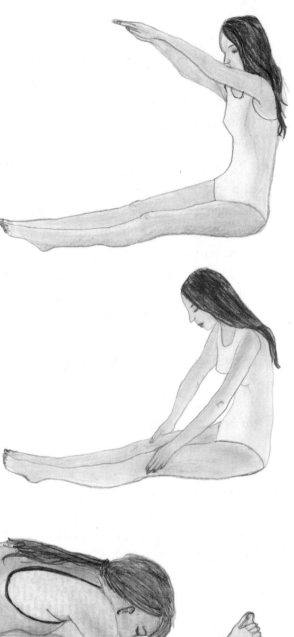

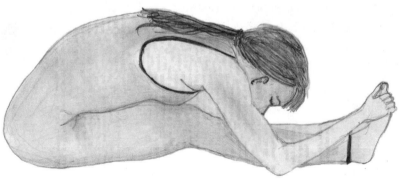

Bent Knee Pose

This posture is similar to the Sitting Head to Knee Pose, and is also done while sitting on the floor. This movement will also tone the internal organs, invigorate the nervous system, and keep the spine supple. In addition, it will stretch your back muscles and help align the vertebra.

Sitting upright on the floor with your legs extended straight out in front, bend your right knee to bring the sole of the right foot flat against the inner left thigh. Inhale while raising both arms parallel and above the head. Keeping the natural curve in the lower part of your back, exhale, relaxing forward, bending from the hips. Keep the left leg straight and reach as far as is comfortable down your leg, even to your foot or beyond. Gently hold your lower leg or toes and draw your chest as close to the top of your thigh as possible, maintaining the natural curve of your lower back while keeping the spine as straight as possible. Relax your neck and shoulders. Do not force your head down. Hold for 30 seconds. Inhale and maintain the stretch while raising your torso back into the upright seated position.

Repeat the Bent Knee Pose with your right knee bent two or three more times.

Switch legs (left knee bent and the sole of your left foot flat against your inner right thigh) and do three more movements.

People with knee problems, lower back problems, high blood pressure, hiatal hernia, inguinal hernia, stomach ulcers, or duodenal ulcers should not do this exercise.

Corpse Pose (again)

Remember to return to the Corpse Pose when finished with the Leg Lift Series and the Sitting Forward Bend Series. Lie quietly on your back, legs extended and about shoulder width apart. Your arms should be extended at about a 45-degree angle, palms relaxed and facing upward. It is fine to have a blanket to lie on and another as a cover. Rest in this position for a few minutes.

CREATING A
Support Network

When dealing with our own health and the health of others, it is wise to build a support network. Loved ones and mentors are the ideal people to include in a support group.

Some members of this network should be our closest family and friends. Build relationships of openness and trust. Encourage honest and compassionate descriptions of each other's health. For a variety of reasons, people are often secretive about their health problems. Sometimes it is because there is an element of denial. Other times information is withheld out of an urge to protect loved ones from worry. Some people do not wish to complain about aches and pains that may be inconsequential. Others are inclined to drift off toward hypochondria, fearing a variety of signals the body is sending. If we have tendencies in any of these directions, honest, straightforward friends can be our best instructors.

We also need people who are steady and have navigated through whatever physical problem we are dealing with. We need to be able to let our hair down. At some point we may need to be that steady support for someone else.

Include a medical professional or mentor in your support network. This easily accessible person must be trustworthy—someone who will listen to what we are saying and will either answer our questions or help us find the answers to those questions. Ideally, people in this capacity will be supportive and nonjudgmental about the course of action we choose. Additionally, they should be positioned to offer advice without expecting anything in return. It is possible for family members to be mentors, if they can be emotionally detached enough to keep their own issues and feelings in check.

The word "mentor" comes from the Indo-European root "men," which means "to think." The original Mentor was really the goddess of wisdom, Athena, who appeared in disguise as a wizened old man offering selfless advice to Telemachas, the son of Odysseus. We want someone like Mentor on our team.

One of the best ways a support network can help is by providing ready access to each other during periods of physical, mental, and emotional stress. Thoughts and emotions have biochemical components. Specific parts of the brain are associated with certain emotions. The same parts of the brain are also associated with specific patterns of hormone regulation.[1] Difficult emotions such as grief, guilt, and fear create toxic chemicals that negatively affect the body.[2] Researchers Brent Q. Hafen, Keith J. Karren, Kathryn J. Frandsen, and N. Lee Smith have noted that people with an optimistic outlook have fewer illnesses and live longer than pessimists.[3] One-quarter of gastroenterology patients suffer from major depression.[4] Marvelously, sharing our feelings with friends helps cleanse the body and lift the spirits. Try it.

Of course attitude is often critical in how well we heal. In recent decades a great deal of empirical evidence has been amassed showing a strong mind-body connection.[5] Some experts who have analyzed this material believe the mind can always fix the body.[6] This has helped many, but it has also created a crisis of guilt and soul searching when a disease continues in spite of strong mental effort. Nevertheless, the hope embodied in the mind-body line of thinking is that we may have greater personal control over our health and healing processes. However, there are times when healing is less about personal control and more about personal surrender.

Simple Cleanse

Health is not an end in itself; it is a means to an end. Health can be a vehicle to serve our larger purpose in life. A healthy body is not the purpose of life. Nobody lives forever. If our only focus is our physical well-being, we may miss the most important parts of life. For many people, reconnecting with their root values, and living deliberately in the service of those values, can be the most powerful way to heal.

Gathering a support group will not only hasten healing, it can give us the power to become involved in important activities and/or social actions outside of ourselves, such as growing a garden, buying organic foods in bulk, or organizing to ban the use of toxic chemicals.

CONCLUSION

The rules are simple: Take care of your body. Pay attention to what you eat. Closely watch your body's signals. Pay attention to what you are thinking. Don't be afraid to face the places that need to be changed. Healing is possible.

If your stomach is bothered after you eat certain types of food, avoid these foods in the future. There are benefits to eating simply, but don't be afraid to explore. Our body's responses will reveal which foods are best suited to our needs.

Exercise. Don't hurt yourself, but do push a little. Take a hike. Hit the yoga mat. We need to find coaches and teachers who understand or are willing to understand our physical situation. See what can be done. We need to surprise ourselves.

This book offers much practical advice that may help to quickly clear up a problem. It also may raise questions and point you in directions to search for additional information. Millions of people may have the same health condition that you have, but even if their solution is similar to yours, we each must explore and take our own personal path to improved health and deep healing.

The most common source of physical suffering for most of us is the abdominal region and the rippling, writhing length of the large intestine.

Not all digestive problems can be prevented or controlled simply with lifestyle changes. Some conditions are hereditary; others are symptoms of infections or other causes, known or unknown. If your symptoms linger or become a daily annoyance, seek out the services of a health care professional. Often problems develop that would have been of little consequence if only they had been treated earlier. Sometimes problems can be avoided altogether just by following a sensible program of cleansing and renewal.

> *May all beings be happy.*
> *May all suffering cease.*
> *May every heart be filled with love.*
> *And may we all know peace.*[1]

NOTES

Introduction to Simple Cleansing

[1] Bernard Jensen, *Dr. Jensen's Guide to Better Bowel Care* (New York: Penguin Putnam Avery, 1999).

[2] Linda Berry, *Internal Cleansing* (New York: Three Rivers Press, 2000).

[3] E. V. Younglai, W. G. Foster, E. G. Hughes, K. Trim, and J. F. Jarrell. "Levels of environmental contaminants in human follicular fluid, serum, and seminal plasma of couples undergoing in vitro fertilization," *Archives of Environmental Contamination and Toxicology* 43, no. 1 (2002): 121–126.

[4] B. Weiss, S. Amler, and R. W. Amler, "Pesticides," *Pediatrics* 113, no. 4 (2004): S1030–S1036. See full text at www.pediatrics.org. See also Pesticide Action Network North America and Commonweal, *Nowhere to Hide: Persistent Toxic Chemicals in the U.S. Food Supply*, (San Francisco: PANNA, 2001).

[5] Weiss, Amler, and Amler, "Pesticides"

[6] Francine Stephens, "Persistent Organic Pollutants: Chemicals That Won't Go Away and Hurt Us All," *Children's Health Environmental Coalition*, November 2002, www.checnet.org/healthehouse/education/articles.asp.

[7] John McDougall, "A Cesspool of Pollutants: Now is the Time to Clean-up Your Body," *McDougall Newsletter*, 3, no. 8 (August 2004).

[8] Berry, *Internal Cleansing*

[9] Younglai et al., "Environmental contaminants in human follicular fluid"

[10] McDougall, "Cesspool of Pollutants"

[11] S. H. Swan, R. L. Kruse, L. Fan, D. B. Barr, E. Z. Drobnis, J. B. Redmon, C. Wang, C. Brazil, J. W. Overstreet, and the Study for the Future of Families Research Group, "Semen quality in relation to biomarkers of pesticide exposure," *Environmental Health Perspectives* 111, no. 12 (2003): 1478–1484.

[12] Berry, *Internal Cleansing*

[13] A. G. Andersen, T. K. Jensen, E. Carlsen, N. Jørgensen, A. M. Andersson, T. Krarup, N. Keiding, and N. E. Skakkebæk, "High frequency of sub-optimal semen quality in an unselected population of young men," *Human Reproduction* 15, no. 2 (2002): 366–372.

[14] S. Irvine, E. Cawood, D. Richardson, E. MacDonald, and J. Aitken, "Evidence of deteriorating semen quality in the United Kingdom: Birth cohort study in 577 men in Scotland over 11 years," *British Medical Journal* 312 (1966): 467-471.

[15] Swan et al., "Semen quality in relation to biomarkers of pesticide exposure"

[16] Berry, *Internal Cleansing*

[17] Weiss, Amler, and Amler, "Pesticides." See also Pesticide Action Network North America, and Commonweal, "Nowhere to Hide."

[18] Y. L. Guo, P. C. Hsu, C. C. Hsu, and G. H. Lambert, "Semen quality after prenatal exposure to polychlorinated biphenyls and dibenzofurans," *Lancet* 356, no. 9237 (2000): 1240–1241.

[19] Sandra Steingraber, "The Benefits of Breast Milk Outweigh Any Risks," CHEC's *HealtheHouse*, May 2002, www.checnet.org/healthehouse/education/articles-detail.asp?Main_ID=451.

[20] Ibid.

[21] Weiss, Amler, and Amler, "Pesticides"

[22] R. Duarte-Davidson and K. C. Jones, "Polychlorinated biphenyls (PCBs) in the UK population: Estimated intake, exposure and body burden," *Science of the Total Environment* 151, no. 2 (1994): 131–152, Summary in National Center for Biotechnology Information (NCBI), National Library of Medicine, ww.ncbi.nlm.nih.gov/entrez/query.

[23] Steingraber, "Benefits of Breast Milk"

[24] McDougall, "Cesspool of Pollutants"

[25] Berry, *Internal Cleansing*

[26] Ibid.

[27] Weiss, Amler, and Amler, "Pesticides"

[28] Sandra Cabot, "Vital Principles," www.weightcontroldoctor.com.

[29] McDougall, "Cesspool of Pollutants"

[30] Ibid.

31 R. J. Gilbert, "Pore-forming toxins," *Cellular and Molecular Life Sciences* 59, no. 5 (2002): 832–844. Abstract available at National Center for Biotechnology Information (NCBI), National Library of Medicine, ww.ncbi.nlm.nih.gov/entrez/query.

32 Doug J. Lisle and Alan Goldhamer, *The Pleasure Trap* (Summertown, TN: Book Publishing Company, 2003).

33 Ibid.

34 Ibid.

35 K. A. Houpt, "Gastrointestinal factors in hunger and satiety," *Neuroscience Biobehavoral Review* 6, no. 2 (1982): 145–164.

36 Lisle and Goldhamer, *Pleasure Trap*

37 Ibid.

38 Ibid.

39 Brenda Davis and Vesanto Melina, *Becoming Vegan* (Summertown, TN: Book Publishing Company, 2000).

40 Ibid.

41 Lisle and Goldhamer, *Pleasure Trap*

42 Vesanto Melina, Brenda Davis, and Victoria Harrison, *Becoming Vegetarian* (Summertown, TN: Book Publishing Company, 2003).

43 Ibid.

44 Ibid.

45 Ibid.

46 Ibid.

47 Berry, *Internal Cleansing*

48 Melina, Davis, and Harrison, *Becoming Vegetarian*

49 Ibid.

50 Raoul Birnbaum, *The Healing Buddha* (Boston: Shambhala, 1989).

51 Jacquelyn W. McClelland, *Your Diet and Cancer* (North Carolina Cooperative Extension Service, Electronic Publication Number HE382, March 1994).

52 Ron Kennedy, "Fats in Nutrition," *The Doctors' Medical Library*, www.medical=library.net/sites/framer.html?/sites/_fats_in_nutrition.html.

53 L. E. Armstrong, "Caffeine, body fluid-electrolyte balance, and exercise performance," *International Journal of Sport Nutrition Exercise and Metabolism* 12, no. 2 (2002): 189–206, National Center for Biotechnology Information (NCBI), National Library of Medicine, www.ncbi.nlm.nih.gov/entrez/query.

54 Mayo Clinic staff, "Unusual urine odor: What does it mean?" *MayoClinic.com*, November 30, 2004, www.mayoclinic.com.

The Digestive Tract

[1] Lynn Marguilis and Dorian Sagan, *Microcosmos* (New York: Touchstone Books, Simon & Schuster, 1986).

[2] Riane Eisler, *The Chalice and the Blade: Our History, Our Future* (New York: HarperCollins, 1988).

[3] Doug J. Lisle and Alan Goldhamer, *The Pleasure Trap* (Summertown, TN: Book Publishing Company, 2003).

[4] Steve Meyerowitz, *Food Combining and Digestion* (Great Barrington, MA: Sproutman Publications, 2002).

[5] Vicky Hallett, "Scents and Sensibility," *U.S. News and World Report*, November 22, 2004.

[6] Raoul Birnbaum, *The Healing Buddha* (Boston: Shambhala, 1989).

[7] Cancer Council of South Australia, "Macrobiotic diets," www.cancersa.org.au (accessed March 3, 2004).

[8] Cynthia Bye, "Reducing your toxic load," www.naturopathic.org/members/development/docs/reducing_toxic_loads.pdf.

[9] B. Q. Hafen, K. J. Karren, K. J. Frandsen, and N. L. Smith, *Mind/Body Health: The Effects of Attitudes, Emotions, and Relationships* (Needham Heights, MA: Allyn and Bacon, 1996).

[10] Peter Gott, "Strange digestive problem is tough to swallow," *Commercial Appeal*, Memphis (TN) November 27, 2004.

[11] American College of Gastroenterology, "The Word on GERD," www.acg.gi.org/patients/gerd/word.asp.

[12] Amanda Spake, *U.S. News and World Report*, Nov 8, 2004 [J. C. Gregor, "Acid suppression and pneumonia: A clinical indication for rational prescribing," *JAMA* 292 (2004): 2012–2013]. Also see Daniel J. DeNoon, "Stomach Acid-Suppressing Drugs May Raise Pneumonia Risk," Fox News Channel, October 26, 2004.

[13] Ibid.

[14] Nancy Touchette, "Pylori Paradox: Microbe Harms Stomach but Protects Esophagus," *Genome News Network*, April 4, 2003.

[15] Sylvia S. Mader, *Biology*, 4th ed. (Dubuque, IA: Wm. C. Brown Publishers, 1993).

[16] Linda Berry, *Internal Cleansing* (New York: Three Rivers Press, 2000).

[17] Paul Talaly and Jed W. Fahey, "Phytochemicals from cruciferous plants protect against cancer by modulating carcinogen metabolism," *American Society for Nutritional Sciences Journal of Nutrition*, 131 (November 2001): S3027–S3033.

[18] Ben Kallen, "Raw, cooked, frozen, or canned?" *Men's Fitness*, September 2002.

[19] Priya Shah, "Food Sources That Boost Glutathione Naturally," *NaturalHealthWeb.com*, first published in *The Glutathione Report*, July 2004, www.glutathione-report.com.

[20] Bye, "Reducing toxic load"

[21] J. M. Samet, "What can we expect from epidemiologic studies of chemical mixtures?" *Toxicology* 105, nos. 2–3 (1995): 307–314.

[22] Healing Edge Sciences, "The Amazing Liver: Liver Disease Risk Factors," www.healingedge.net/cat_liver.html. Updated December 27, 2003.

[23] Sandra Cabot, "Vital Principles," www.weightcontroldoctor.com.

[24] Cathy Wong, "Arginine," www.about.com.

[25] Cabot, "Vital Principles"

[26] "Methionine: What is it?" www.wholehealthmd.com.

[27] Vesanto Melina and Michael Klaper, "Creating and Maintaining a Healthy Intestinal Boundary," in Vesanto Melina, Jo Stepaniak, and Dina Aronson, *Food Allergy Survival Guide* (Summertown, TN: Healthy Living Publications, Book Publishing Company, 2004).

[28] Mayo Foundation for Medical Education and Research, www.mayoclinic.com.

[29] Ibid.

[30] D. Kritchevsky, S. A. Tepper, and D. M. Klurfeld, "Effect of pectin and cellulose on formation and regression of gallstones in hamsters," *Experientia*, 40, no. 4 (1984): 350–351.

[31] Charles B. Clayton, *The American Medical Association Family Medical Guide* (New York: Random House, 1994).

[32] C. Morton, A. L. Klatsky, and N. Udaltsova, "Smoking, coffee, and pancreatitis," *American Journal of Gastroenterology* 99, no. 4 (2004): 731.

[33] Melina and Klaper, "Intestinal Boundary"

[34] Elizabeth Lipski, *Digestive Wellness* (Los Angeles: Keats Publishing, 2000).

[35] Ibid.

[36] Ibid.

The Large Intestine: Problems and Solutions

[1] The Editors of *Consumer Reports*, *The Medicine Show* (Mount Vernon, NY: Consumers Union, 1974).

[2] Anissa Anderson Orr, "Camera pill reveals 'inside' story on pain relievers," *Findings at Baylor College of Medicine, Houston, Texas,* www.bcmfindings.net/vol1/is6/03june_n1.htm.

[3] N. Somchit, F. Sanat, E. H. Gan, A. W. Shahrin, and A. Zuraini, "Liver injury induced by the non-steroidal anti-inflammatory drug mefenamic acid," *Singapore Medical Journal* 45, no. 11(2004): 530.

[4] Mayo Foundation for Medical Education and Research, www.mayoclinic.com.

[5] Orr, "Camera pill"

[6] "Pain Pills Cause Hidden Damage," *Prevention,* November 2003.

[7] Mayo Clinic staff, "NSAIDs: How to avoid side effects," (function test abnormalities) MayoClinic.com *Pain Management Center,* www.mayoclinic.com (accessed February 1, 2005). See also Somchit et al., "Liver injury" (elevation of liver enzymes to severe hepatic necrosis).

[8] M. S. Micozzi, C. L. Carter, D. Albanes, P. R. Taylor, and L. M. Licitra (Armed Forces Institute of Pathology), "Bowel function and breast cancer in US women," *American Journal of Public Health* 79, no. 1(1989): 73–75, www.ajph.org/cgi/content/abstract/79/1/73.

[9] N. L. Petrakis and E. B. King, "Cytological abnormalities in nipple aspirates of breast fluid from women with severe constipation," *Lancet* 2, no. 8257 (1981): 1203–1204.

[10] Nicholas L. Petrakis, MD, quoted in "Constipation and Breast Cancer," *Saturday Evening Post,* April 1982.

[11] Bernard Jensen and Sylvia Bell, *Tissue Cleansing Through Bowel Management* (Escondido, CA: Bernard Jensen, DC, 1981).

[12] John Harvey Kellogg quoted in "Better health by cleansing," http://hps-online.com.

[13] John McDougall, "Hemorrhoids, Varicose Veins, The McDougall Program: Diet and Lifestyle Implications," www.drmcdougall.com/science/constipation.html.

[14] Stephen Barrett, MD, "Gastrointestinal Quackery: Colonics, Laxatives, and More," Quackwatch Home Page, www.quackwatch.org (accessed March 2004).

[15] Editors *Consumer Reports, Medicine Show*

[16] Sandra Cabot, "Vital Principles," www.weightcontroldoctor.com.

[17] Gayle Reichler and Nancy Burke, *Active Wellness* (New York: Time Life Books, 1998).

[18] Rossella Lorenzi, "Martin Luther's Toilet Flushed Out," *Discovery News,* (accessed February 1, 2005). http://dsc.discovery.com/news/briefs/20041025/luther.html.

[19] "Luther's lavatory thrills experts," *BBC News World Edition,* Friday, October 22, 2004, http://news.bbc.co.uk/2/hi/europe/3944549.stm.

[20] Harish Johari, "Pearls of Wisdom—Harish Johari on Health," interview by Carrie Angus, MD, February/March 1997, http://sanatansociety.org/.

[21] Swami Vishnudevananda, *The Complete Illustrated Book of Yoga* (New York: Julian Press, 1960).

[22] Benjamin Spock and Steven J. Parker, *Dr. Spock's Baby and Child Care*, 8th ed. (New York: Simon & Schuster, 1998).

[23] Ibid.

[24] Editors of *Consumer Reports, Medicine Show*

[25] McDougall, "McDougall Program"

[26] Ibid.

[27] National Council Against Health Fraud (NCAHF), "NCAHF Position Paper on Colonic Irrigation," NCAHF, PO Box 1276, Loma Linda, CA 92354-1276.

[28] Barrett, "Gastrointestinal Quackery"

[29] International Association for Colon Hydrotherapy, "Historical view," PO Box 461285, San Antonio, TX 78246-1285, http://I-ACT.org.

[30] Editors of *Consumer Reports, The Medicine Show*

[31] NCAHF, "Position Paper"

[32] U.S. Food and Drug Administration, "Most recent warning letters," www.fda.gov. See also U.S. Food and Drug Administration, Center for Devices and Radiological Health, www.fda.gov/cdrh.

[33] G. Gayer, R. Zissin, S. Apter, A. Oscadchy, and M. Hertz, "Perforations of the rectosigmoid colon induced by cleansing enema: CT findings in 14 patients," *Abdominal Imaging* 27, no. 4 (2002): 453–457.

[34] Barrett, "Gastrointestinal Quackery"

[35] E. Ernst, "Colonic irrigation and the theory of autointoxication: A triumph of ignorance over science," *Journal of Clinical Gastroenterology* 24, no. 4 (1997): 196–198.

[36] Ibid.

[37] Jensen and Bell, *Tissue Cleansing*

[38] Barrett, "Gastrointestinal Quackery"

[39] M. Lemann, B. Flourie, L. Picon, B. Coffin, R. Jian, and J. C. Rambaud, "Motor activity recorded in the unprepared colon of healthy humans," *Gut* 37, no. 5 (1995): 649–653. http://gut.bmjjournals.com/cgi/content/abstract/37/5/649.

[40] Editors of *Consumer Reports, Medicine Show*

[41] NCAHF, "Position Paper"

[42] Ibid.

[43] Barrett, "Gastrointestinal Quackery"

[44] Arthur C. Guyton, "Disorders of the Large Intestine," in *Textbook of Medical Physiology*, 9th ed. (Philadelphia: W. B. Sounders Company, 1996).

[45] B. Q. Hafen, K. J. Karren, K. J. Frandsen, and N. L. Smith, *Mind/Body Health: The Effects of Attitudes, Emotions, and Relationships* (Needham Heights, MA: Allyn and Bacon, 1996).

[46] University of Pittsburgh Medical Center, "Irritable Bowel Syndrome: Treatment Options," http://irritablebowel.upmc.com/treatment.htm.

[47] McKinley Health Center, "Irritable Bowel Syndrome," *Cecil's Textbook of Information*, 21st ed. (Urbana-Champaign: University of Illinois, 2000), www.mckinley.uiuc.edu/handouts/irr-bowe/irr-bowe.html.

[48] W. M. Gonsalkorale and P. J. Whorwell, "Hypnotherapy in the treatment of irritable bowel syndrome," *European Journal of Gastroenterology and Hepatology* 17, no. 1 (2005): 15–20.

[49] W. M. Gonsalkorale, V. Miller, A. Afzal, and P. J. Whorwell, "Long-term benefits of hypnotherapy for irritable bowel syndrome," *Gut* 52, no. 11 (2003): 1623–1629.

[50] Vesanto Melina and Michael Klaper, "Creating and Maintaining a Healthy Intestinal Boundary," in Vesanto Melina, Jo Stepaniak, and Dina Aronson, *Food Allergy Survival Guide* (Summertown, TN: Healthy Living Publications, Book Publishing Company, 2004).

[51] Bryanna Clark Grogan, "Fiber: What's it all about?" in *The Fiber for Life Cookbook* (Summertown, TN: Book Publishing Company, 2002).

[52] Melina and Klaper, "Intestinal Boundary"

[53] Karen L. Schneider, "How Clean Should Your Colon Be?" *Council on Science and Health*, February 27, 2003.

[54] UNICEF, *The State of the World's Children 1998,* (Oxfordshire, UK: Oxford University Press, 1998).

[55] Ibid.

[56] Lauran Neergaard, "Maggots make medical comeback for wound healing," Associated Press, *Daily Herald,* Columbia (TN) August 3, 2004.

[57] UNICEF, *World's Children*

[58] Jay W. Marks, "Giardiasis," *MedicineNet.com,* March 22, 2005, www.medicinenet.com/giardia_lamblia/article.htm.

[59] Centers for Disease Control National Center for Infectious Diseases, "Shigella," September 3, 2003, www.cdc.gov/ncidod/dbmd/diseaseinfo/shigellosis_g.htm.

[60] Ibid.

[61] BMC Public Health, "Overweight, obesity and colorectal cancer screening: Disparity between men and women," November 8, 2004, www.biomedcentral.com/1471=2458/4/.

[62] Hali Wickner, "Cancer prevention, calcium and vitamin D," Dartmouth Medical School, January 12, 2004, study originally reported in *Journal of the National Cancer Institute*, December 3, 2003, www.dartmouth.edu/~vox/0304/0112/nutrients.html.

[63] Ibid.

[64] "It takes two to fight colon cancer," *Prevention*, June 2004.

[65] Cynthia Floyd Manley, "Direct link found between chronic inflammation, colon cancer," Vanderbilt Medical Center, *The Reporter*, November 7, 2003. See also Joanna Downer, "Inflammation marker predicts colon cancer," *Johns Hopkins Medicine News and Information Services*, February 3, 2004.

[66] Christine Gorman and Alice Park, "The Fires Within," *Time*, February 23, 2004.

[67] Manley, "Chronic inflammation"

[68] Gorman and Park, "Fires Within"

[69] Ibid.

[70] Ibid.

[71] Jane E. Brody, "Can an Aspirin a Day Keep the Doctor Away?" in *The World Book Year Book* (Chicago: World Book-Childcraft International, 1981).

[72] Ibid.

[73] Gorman and Park, "Fires Within"

[74] Deborah Kimbell, "An Aspirin a Day May Keep Colon Cancer Away, Dartmouth Researchers Find," *Dartmouth Medical School News*, March 5, 2003.

[75] Joanna Downer, "Inflammation marker"

[76] National Cancer Institute, "NCI-Sponsored Trials of Cyclooxygenase (COX) Inhibitors for Cancer Prevention and Treatment," December 17, 2004, www.nci.nih.gov/newscenter/COXInhibitorsFactSheet. See also Gorman and Park, "Fires Within."

[77] Associated Press, "FDA urges alternatives to Celebrex," December 18, 2004, www.msnbc.msn.com/id/6727955/. For more information about regulation of COX-2 inhibitors by the FDA, visit the FDA Web site at www.fda.gov/cder/drug/.

[78] D. A. Snowdon and R. L. Phillips, "Coffee consumption and risk of fatal cancers," *American Journal of Public Health* 74, no. 8 (1984): 820–823.

[79] A. Tavani and C. La Vecchia, "Coffee, decaffeinated coffee, tea and cancer of the colon and rectum: A review of epidemiological studies, 1990–2003," *Cancer Causes and Control* 15, no. 8 (2004): 743–757. National Center for Biotechnology Information (NCBI), National Library of Medicine. See also C. G. Woolcott, W. D. King, and L. D. Marrett, "Coffee and tea consumption and cancers of the bladder, colon and rectum," *European Journal of Cancer Prevention* 11, no. 2 (2002): 137–145; E. Giovannucci, "Meta-analysis of coffee consumption and risk of colorectal cancer," *American Journal of Epidemiology* 147, no. 11 (1998): 1043–1052.

[80] Tavani and La Vecchia, "Review of epidemiological studies"

[81] Giovannucci, "Coffee consumption risk"

[82] A. T. Fleischauer, C. Poole, and L. Arab, "Garlic consumption and cancer prevention: Meta-analyses of colorectal and stomach cancers," *American Journal of Clinical Nutrition* 72, no. 4 (2000): 1047–1052.

[83] A. T. Fleischauer and L. Arab, "Garlic and cancer: A critical review of the epidemiologic literature," *Journal of Nutrition* 131, no. 3 (2001): S1032–S1040.

[84] M. S. Sandhu, I. R. White, and K. McPherson, "Systematic review of the prospective cohort studies on meat consumption and colorectal cancer risk: A meta-analytical approach," *Cancer Epidemiology, Biomarkers, and Prevention* 10, no. 5 (2001): 439–446.

[85] E. Riboli and T. Norat, "Epidemiologic evidence of the protective effect of fruit and vegetables on cancer risk," *American Journal of Clinical Nutrition* 78, no. 3 (2003): S559–S569.

[86] T. J. Key, A. Schatzkin, W. C. Willett, N. E. Allen, E. A. Spencer, and R. C. Travis, "Diet, nutrition and the prevention of cancer," *Public Health and Nutrition* 7, no. 2 (2004): 187–200.

[87] M. L. Slattery, K. P. Curtin, S. L. Edwards, and D. M. Schaffer, "Plant foods, fiber, and rectal cancer," *American Journal of Clinical Nutrition*, 79, no. 2 (2004): 274–281.

[88] Gloria McVeigh, "Fiber fights rectal cancer," *Prevention*, August 2004.

[89] Ibid.

[90] Linda Berry, *Internal Cleansing* (New York: Three Rivers Press, 2000).

[91] Mayo Foundation for Medical Education and Research, www.mayoclinic.com.

[92] Vesanto Melina, Brenda Davis, and Victoria Harrison, *Becoming Vegetarian* (Summertown, TN: Book Publishing Company, 2003).

[93] Berry, *Internal Cleansing*

[94] Bonnie Liebman, "Ten Myths That Won't Quit," *Nutrition Action Health Letter, Center for Science in the Public Interest* 31, no. 10 (December 2004).

95 C. M. Friedenreich and M. R. Orenstein, "Physical activity and cancer prevention: Etiologic evidence and biological mechanisms," *Journal of Nutrition* 132, no. 11 (2002): S3456–S3464.

96 Key et al., "Diet, nutrition"

97 BMC Public Health, "Obesity and colorectal cancer"

The Weekend Cleanse Plan

1 Doug J. Lisle and Alan Goldhamer, *The Pleasure Trap* (Summertown, TN: Book Publishing Company, 2003).

2 American Academy of Family Physicians, "Bacterial Endocarditis: A heart at risk," familydoctor.org, American Academy of Family Physicians, from "Management of Bacterial Endocarditis," *American Family Physician*, March 15, 2000, www.aafp.org/afp/2000315/1725.html.

3 Linda Berry, *Internal Cleansing* (New York: Three Rivers Press, 2000).

4 Mayo Foundation for Medical Education and Research, "Sweating and Body Odor," December 9, 2004, www.mayoclinic.com.

5 Dean Falk, "Constraints on brain size: The radiator hypothesis," in *The Evolution of Primate Nervous Systems* ed. Todd M. Preuss and Jon H. Kaas, vol. 5, *Evolution of Nervous Systems*, ed. Jon Kaas et al. (forthcoming Elsevier–Academic Press), www.anthro.fsu.edu/people/faculty/falk/radpapweb.htm.

6 Steve Meyerowitz, *Juice Fasting and Detoxification* (Great Barrington, MA: Sproutman Publications, 1999).

7 Berry, *Internal Cleansing*

8 Martin Stone, "Lemon Balm," *Making Scents,* Summer/Fall 2004, from *Herbs Explained* by Martin Stone (Bloomington, IN: AuthorHouse, 2003).

9 Berry, *Internal Cleansing*

10 Sharon Gillson, "Heartburn/Acid Reflux," http://heartburn.about.com/od/understandingheartburn/a/heartburn_facts.htm.

11 Karen Blum, "Coffee raises blood pressure, though not by much," *Johns Hopkins Medicine News and Information Services*, March 25, 2002, http://www.hopkinsmedicine.org/press/2002/MARCH/020324.htm; M. J. Klag, N. Wang, L. A. Brancati, L. A. Cooper, K. Liang, J. H. Young, and D. E. Ford, "Coffee intake and the risk of hypetension," *Archives of Internal Medicine* 162 (March 2002): 657–662. On the increased possibility of urinary tract cancer, see M. P. Zeegers, F. E. Tan, R. A. Goldbohm, and P. A. van den Brandt, "Are coffee and tea consumption associated with urinary tract cancer risk? A systematic review and meta-analysis,"

International Journal of Epidemiology 30, no. 2 (2001): 353–362. See also D. A. Snowdon and R. L. Phillips, "Coffee consumption and risk of fatal cancers," *American Journal of Public Health* 74, no. 8 (1984): 820–823.

[12] Blum, "Coffee raises blood pressure"

[13] I. Kawachi, G. A. Colditz, and C. B. Stone, "Does coffee drinking increase the risk of coronary heart disease? Results from a meta-analysis," *British Heart Journal* 72, no. 3 (1994): 269–275.

[14] P. C. Pozniak, "The carcinogenicity of caffeine and coffee: A review," *Journal of the American Dietary Association* 85, no. 9 (1985): 1127–1133.

[15] Zeegers et al., "Urinary tract cancer risk"

[16] Berry, *Internal Cleasing*

[17] Meyerowitz, *Juice Fasting*

[18] Ibid.

[19] Steve Meyerowitz, *Food Combining and Digestion* (Great Barrington, MA: Sproutman Publications, 2002).

[20] Ibid.

[21] Mayo Foundation for Medical Education and Research, www.mayoclinic.com.

[22] J. W. Shields, "Lymph, lymph glands, and homeostasis," *Lymphology* 25, no. 4 (December 1992): 147–153, NCBI National Library of Medicine.

[23] Ram Das, "Cookbook for a sacred life," in *Be Here Now* (San Cristobal, NM: Lama Foundation, 1971).

[24] Healing Edge Sciences, "The Amazing Liver: Liver Disease Risk Factors," www.healingedge.net/store.html. Updated December 27, 2003.

Exercise

[1] The Editors of *Consumer Reports*, *The Medicine Show* (Mount Vernon, NY: Consumers Union, 1974).

[2] Bernard Jensen, *Dr. Jensen's Guide to Better Bowel Care* (New York: Penguin Putnam Avery, 1999).

Creating a Support Network

[1] B. Q. Hafen, K. J. Karren, K. J. Frandsen, and N. L. Smith, *Mind/Body Health: The Effects of Attitudes, Emotions, and Relationships* (Needham Heights, MA: Allyn and Bacon, 1996).

[2] Berry, *Internal Cleasing*

[3] Hafen et al., *Mind/Body Health*

[4] Ibid.

[5] Cheryl Townsley, "Unresolved emotions," in *Cleansing Made Simple* (Littleton, CO: LFH Publishing, 2001).

[6] Louise L. Hays, *Heal Your Body* (Carson, CA: Hay House, 1988).

Conclusion

[1] Kathryn Hutchens, January 2005.

SOURCES

Books

Berry, Linda. *Internal Cleansing*. New York: Three Rivers Press, 2000.

Birnbaum, Raoul. *The Healing Buddha*. Boston: Shambhala, 1989.

Burroughs, Stanley. *The Master Cleanser*. Reno: Burroughs Books, 1993.

Clayton, Charles B. *The American Medical Association Family Medical Guide*. New York: Random House, 1994.

Consumer Reports, eds. *The Medicine Show*. Mount Vernon, NY: Consumers Union, 1974.

Das, Ram. *Be Here Now*. San Cristobal, NM: Lama Foundation, 1971.

Davis, Brenda, and Vesanto Melina. *Becoming Vegan*. Summertown, TN: Book Publishing Company, 2000.

Eisler, Riane. *The Chalice and the Blade: Our History, Our Future*. New York: HarperCollins, 1988.

Grogan, Bryanna Clark. *The Fiber for Life Cookbook*. Summertown, TN: Book Publishing Company, 2002.

Guyton, Arthur C. *Textbook of Medical Physiology*. 9th ed. Philadelphia: W. B. Sounders Company, 1996.

Hafen, B. Q., K. J. Karren, K. J. Frandsen, and N. L. Smith. *Mind/Body Health: The Effects of Attitudes, Emotions, and Relationships*. Needham Heights, MA: Allyn and Bacon, 1996.

Hays, Louise L. *Heal Your Body*. Carson, CA: Hay House 1988.

Jensen, Bernard. *Dr. Jensen's Guide to Better Bowel Care*. New York: Penguin Putnam Avery, 1999.

Jensen, Bernard, and Sylvia Bell. *Tissue Cleansing Through Bowel Management*. Escondido, CA: Bernard Jensen, DC, 1981.

Lisle, Doug J., and Alan Goldhamer. *The Pleasure Trap*. Summertown, TN: Book Publishing Company, 2003.

Lipski, Elizabeth. *Digestive Wellness*. Los Angeles: Keats Publishing, 2000.

Mader, Sylvia S. *Biology*. 4th ed. Dubuque, IA: Wm. C. Brown Publishers, 1993.

Marguilis, Lynn, and Dorian Sagan. *Microcosmos*. New York: Touchstone Books, Simon & Schuster, 1986.

McClelland, Jacquelyn W. *Your Diet and Cancer*. North Carolina Cooperative Extension Service, Electronic Publication Number HE382, March 1994.

Melina, Vesanto, Brenda Davis, and Victoria Harrison. *Becoming Vegetarian*. Summertown, TN: Book Publishing Company, 2003.

Melina, Vesanto, Jo Stepaniak, and Dina Aronson. *Food Allergy Survival Guide*. Summertown, TN: Healthy Living Publications, Book Publishing Company, 2004.

Meyerowitz, Steve. *Food Combining and Digestion*. Great Barrington, MA: Sproutman Publications, 2002.

———. *Juice Fasting and Detoxification*. Great Barrington, MA: Sproutman Publications, 1999.

Reichler, Gayle, and Nancy Burke. *Active Wellness*. New York: Time Life Books, 1998.

Spock, Benjamin, and Steven J. Parker. *Dr. Spock's Baby and Child Care*. 8th ed. New York: Simon & Schuster, 1998.

Townsley, Cheryl. *Cleansing Made Simple*. Littleton, CO: LFH Publishing, 2001.

UNICEF. *The State of the World's Children 1998*. Oxfordshire, UK: Oxford University Press, 1998.

Vishnudevananda, Swami. *The Complete Illustrated Book of Yoga*. New York: Julian Press, 1960.

Articles, Periodicals, and Special Reports

American Academy of Family Physicians. "Bacterial Endocarditis: A heart at risk." familydoctor.org, *American Academy of Family Physicians.* From "Management of Bacterial Endocarditis." *American Family Physician,* March 15, 2000. www.aafp.org/afp/2000315/1725.html.

American College of Gastroenterology. "The Word on GERD." www.acg.gi.org/patients/gerd/word.asp.

Andersen, A. G., T. K. Jensen, E. Carlsen, N. Jørgensen, A. M. Andersson, T. Krarup, N. Keiding, and N. E. Skakkebæk. "High frequency of sub-optimal semen quality in an unselected population of young men." *Human Reproduction* 15, no. 2 (2000): 366-372.

Anderson Orr, Anissa. "Camera pill reveals 'inside' story on pain relievers." *Findings at Baylor College of Medicine, Houston, Texas.* www.bcm.edu/findings.net/vol1/ is6/03june_n1.htm.

Armstrong, L. E. "Caffeine, body fluid-electrolyte balance, and exercise performance." *International Journal of Sport Nutrition Exercise and Metabolism* 12, no. 2 (2002): 189–206. National Center for Biotechnology Information (NCBI), National Library of Medicine. www.ncbi.nlm.nih.gov/entrez/query.

Associated Press. "FDA urges alternatives to Celebrex." December 18, 2004. www.msnbc.msn.com/id/6727955/.

Barrett, Stephen. "Gastrointestinal Quackery: Colonics, Laxatives, and More." Quackwatch Home Page. www.quackwatch.org. (accessed March 2004).

BBC News. "Luther's lavatory thrills experts." *BBC News World Edition,* Friday, October 22, 2004. http://news.bbc.co.uk/2/hi/europe/3944549.stm.

Biomed Central, BMC Public Health. "Overweight, obesity and colorectal cancer screening: Disparity between men and women." November 8, 2004. www.biomedcentral.com/1471–2458/4/.

Blum, Karen. "Coffee raises blood pressure, though not by much," *John Hopkins Medicine News and Information Services,* March 25, 2002. http://www.hopkinsmedicine. org/press/2002/MARCH/020324.htm.

Brody, Jane E. "Can an Aspirin a Day Keep the Doctor Away?" In *The World Book Year Book.* Chicago: World Book-Childcraft International, 1981.

Bye, Cynthia. "Reducing your toxic load." www.naturopathic.org/members/development/docs/reducing_toxic_loads.pdf.

Cabot, Sandra. "Vital Principles." www.weightcontroldoctor.com.

Cancer Council of South Australia. "Macrobiotic diets." www.cancersa.org.au/i-cms?page=1.2.546.562 (accessed March 3, 2004).

Centers for Disease Control National Center for Infectious Diseases. "Shigella." September 3, 2003. www.cdc.gov/ncidod/dbmd/diseaseinfo/shigellosis_g.htm.

DeNoon, Daniel J. "Stomach Acid-Suppressing Drugs May Raise Pneumonia Risk." Fox News Channel, October 26, 2004.

Downer, Joanna. "Inflammation marker predicts colon cancer." *Johns Hopkins Medicine News and Information Services*, February 3, 2004.

Duarte-Davidson, R., and K. C. Jones. "Polychlorinated biphenyls (PCBs) in the UK population: Estimated intake, exposure and body burden." *Science of the Total Environment* 151, no. 2(1994): 131–152. Summary in National Center for Biotechnology Information (NCBI), National Library of Medicine, www.ncbi.nlm.nih.gov/entrez/query.

Ernst, E. "Colonic irrigation and the theory of autointoxication: A triumph of ignorance over science." *Journal of Clinical Gastroenterology* 24, no. 4 (1997): 196-198.

Falk, Dean. "Constraints on brain size: The radiator hypothesis." In *The Evolution of Primate Nervous Systems*, edited by Todd M. Preuss and Jon H. Kaas. *Evolution of Nervous Systems*, forthcoming. Jon Kaas et al. Elsevier–Academic Press. www.anthro.fsu.edu/people/faculty/falk/radpapweb.htm.

Fleischauer, A. T., and L. Arab. "Garlic and cancer: A critical review of the epidemiologic literature." *Journal of Nutrition* 131, no. 3 (2001): S1032–S1040.

Fleischauer, A. T., C. Poole, and L. Arab. "Garlic consumption and cancer prevention: Meta-analyses of colorectal and stomach cancers." *American Journal of Clinical Nutrition* 72, no. 4 (2000): 1047–1052.

Food and Drug Administration. www.fda.gov/cder/drug/.

Friedenreich, C. M., and M. R. Orenstein. "Physical activity and cancer prevention: Etiologic evidence and biological mechanisms." *Journal of Nutrition* 132, no. 11 (2002): S3456–S3464.

Gayer, G., R. Zissin, S. Apter, A. Oscadchy, and M. Hertz. "Perforations of the rectosigmoid colon induced by cleansing enema: CT findings in 14 patients." *Abdominal Imaging* 27, no. 4 (2002): 453–457.

Gilbert, R. J. "Pore-forming toxins." *Cellular and Molecular Life Sciences* 59, no. 5 (2002): 832–844. Abstract available at National Center for Biotechnology Information (NCBI), National Library of Medicine, ww.ncbi.nlm.nih.gov/entrez/query.

Gillson, Sharon. "Heartburn/Acid Reflux." http://heartburn.about.com/od/understandingheartburn/a/heartburn_facts.htm.

Giovannucci, E. "Meta-analysis of coffee consumption and risk of colorectal cancer." *American Journal of Epidemiology* 147, no. 11 (1998): 1043–1052.

Gonsalkorale, W. M., V. Miller, A. Afzal, and P. J. Whorwell. "Long-term benefits of hypnotherapy for irritable bowel syndrome." *Gut* 52, no. 11 (2003): 1623–1629.

Gonsalkorale, W. M., and P. J. Whorwell. "Hypnotherapy in the treatment of irritable bowel syndrome." *European Journal of Gastroenterology and Hepatology* 17, no. 1 (2005): 15–20.

Gorman, Christine, and Alice Park. "The Fires Within." *Time*, February 23, 2004.

Gott, Peter. "Strange digestive problem is tough to swallow." *Commercial Appeal*, Memphis (TN) November 27, 2004.

Guo, Y. L., P. C. Hsu, C. C. Hsu, and G. H. Lambert. "Semen quality after prenatal exposure to polychlorinated biphenyls and dibenzofurans." *Lancet* 356, no. 9237 (2000): 1249-1241.

Hallett, Vicky. "Scents and Sensibility." *U.S. News and World Report*, November 22, 2004.

Healing Edge Sciences. "The Amazing Liver: Liver Disease Risk Factors." www.healingedge.net/store/page187.html. Updated December 27, 2003.

Houpt, K. A. "Gastrointestinal factors in hunger and satiety." *Neuroscience Biobehavoral Review* 6, no. 2 (1982): 145–164.

International Association for Colon Hydrotherapy. "Historical view." PO Box 461285, San Antonio, TX 78246-1285, http://I-ACT.org.

Irvine, S., E. Cawood, D. Richardson, E. MacDonald, and J. Aitken. "Evidence of deteriorating semen quality in the United Kingdom: Birth cohort study in 577 men in Scotland over 11 years." *British Medical Journal* 132 (1966): 467–471.

Johari, Harish. "Pearls of Wisdom–Harish Johari on Health." Interview by Carrie Angus, MD, February/March 1997. http://sanatansociety.org/ayurveda_home_remedies.

Kallen, Ben. "Raw, cooked, frozen, or canned?" *Men's Fitness*, September 2002.

Kawachi, I., G. A. Colditz, and C. B. Stone. "Does coffee drinking increase the risk of coronary heart disease? Results from a meta-analysis," *British Heart Journal* 72, no. 3 (1994): 269–275.

Kellogg, John Harvey, quoted in "Better health by cleansing." http://hps-online.com.

Kennedy, Ron. "Fats in Nutrition," *The Doctors' Medical Library*. www.medical-library.net/sites/sites/_fats_in_nutritiona.html.

Key, T. J., A. Schatzkin, W. C. Willett, N. E. Allen, E. A. Spencer, and R. C. Travis. "Diet, nutrition and the prevention of cancer." *Public Health and Nutrition* 7, no. 1A (2004): 187–200.

Kimbell, Deborah. "An Aspirin a Day May Keep Colon Cancer Away, Dartmouth Researchers Find." *Dartmouth Medical School News*, March 5, 2003.

Klag, M. J., N. Wang, L. A. Meoni, F. L. Brancati, L. A. Cooper, K. Liang, J. H. Young, and D. E. Ford. "Coffee intake and the risk of hypertension," *Archives of Internal Medicine* 162 (March 2002): 657–662.

Kritchevsky, D., S. A. Tepper, and D. M. Klurfeld. "Effect of pectin and cellulose on formation and regression of gallstones in hamsters." *Experientia.* 40, no. 4 (1984): 350–351.

Lemann, M., B. Flourie, L. Picon, B. Coffin, R. Jian, and J. C. Rambaud. "Motor activity recorded in the unprepared colon of healthy humans." *Gut* 37, no. 5 (1995): 649–653. http://gut.bmjjournals.com/cgi/content/abstract/37/5/649.

Liebman, Bonnie. "Ten Myths That Won't Quit." *Nutrition Action Health Letter, Center for Science in the Public Interest* 31, no. 10. (December 2004).

Lorenzi, Rossella. "Martin Luther's Toilet Flushed Out." *Discovery News* (accessed February 1, 2005). http://dsc.discovery.com/news/briefs/20041025/luther.html.

Manley, Cynthia Floyd. "Direct link found between chronic inflammation, colon cancer." Vanderbilt Medical Center, *The Reporter*, November 7, 2003.

Marks, Jay W. "Giardiasis." *MedicineNet.com*, March 22, 2005. www.medicinenet.com/giardia_lamblia/article.htm.

Mayo Clinic staff. "NSAIDs: How to avoid side effects." *MayoClinic.com Pain Management Center.* www.mayoclinic.com. (accessed February 1, 2005).

———. "Unusual urine odor: What does it mean?" *MayoClinic.com*, November 30, 2004. www.mayoclinic.com.

Mayo Foundation for Medical Education and Research. "Sweating and Body Odor." December 9, 2004. www.mayoclinic.com.

McDougall, John. "A Cesspool of Pollutants: Now is the Time to Clean-up Your Body." *McDougall Newsletter* 3, no. 8 (August 2004).

———. "Hemorrhoids, Varicose Veins, The McDougall Program: Diet and Lifestyle Implications." www.drmcdougall.com/science/constipation.html.

McKinley Health Center. "Irritable Bowel Syndrome," *Cecil's Textbook of Information*, 21st ed. Urbana-Champaign: University of Illinois, 2000. www.mckinley.uiuc.edu/handouts/irr=bowe/irr=bowe.html.

McVeigh, Gloria. "Fiber fights rectal cancer." *Prevention*, August 2004.

Micozzi, M. S., C. L. Carter, D. Albanes, P. R. Taylor, and L. M. Licitra (Armed Forces Institute of Pathology). "Bowel function and breast cancer in US women." *American Journal of Public Health* 79, no. 1 (1989): 73–75. www.ajph.org/cgi/content/abstract/79/1/73.

Morton, C., A. L. Klatsky, and N. Udaltsova. "Smoking, coffee, and pancreatitis." *American Journal of Gastroenterology* 99, no. 4 (2004): 731.

National Cancer Institute. "NCI-Sponsored Trials of Cyclooxygenase (COX) Inhibitors for Cancer Prevention and Treatment." December 17, 2004. www.nci.nih.gov/newscenter/COXInhibitorsFactSheet.

National Council Against Health Fraud (NCAHF). "NCAHF Position Paper on Colonic Irrigation." NCAHF, PO Box 1276, Loma Linda, CA 92354-1276.

Neergaard, Lauran. "Maggots make medical comeback for wound healing." Associated Press, *Daily Herald*, Columbia (TN) August 3, 2004.

Pesticide Action Network North America and Commonweal. *Nowhere to Hide: Persistent Toxic Chemicals in the U.S. Food Supply.* San Francisco: PANNA, 2001.

Petrakis, Nicholas L., quoted in "Constipation and Breast Cancer." *Saturday Evening Post*, April 1982.

Petrakis, N. L., and E. B. King. "Cytological abnormalities in nipple aspirates of breast fluid from women with severe constipation." *Lancet* 85, no. 9 (1981): 1203–1204.

Pozniak, P. C. "The carcinogenicity of caffeine and coffee: A review." *Journal of the American Dietary Association* 85, no. 9 (1985): 1127–1133.

Riboli, E., and T. Norat. "Epidemiologic evidence of the protective effect of fruit and vegetables on cancer risk." *American Journal of Clinical Nutrition* 78, no. 3 (2003): S559–S569.

Samet, J. M. "What can we expect from epidemiologic studies of chemical mixtures?" *Toxicology* 105, nos. 2–3 (1995): 307–314.

Sandhu, M. S., I. R. White, and K. McPherson. "Systematic review of the prospective cohort studies on meat consumption and colorectal cancer risk: A meta-analytical approach" *Cancer Epidemiology, and Biomarkers Prevention* 10, no. 5 (2001): 439–446.

Schneider, Karen L. "How Clean Should Your Colon Be?" *Council on Science and Health*, February 27, 2003.

Shah, Priya. "Food Sources That Boost Glutathione Naturally." *NaturalHealthWeb.com*, first published in *The Glutathione Report*, July 2004, www.glutathione-report.com.

Shields, J. W. "Lymph, lymph glands, and homeostasis." *Lymphology*. 25, no. 4 (1992): 147–153. NCBI National Library of Medicine.

Slattery, M. L., K. P. Curtin, S. L. Edwards, and D. M. Schaffer. "Plant foods, fiber, and rectal cancer." *American Journal of Clinical Nutrition* 79, no. 2 (2004): 274–281.

Snowdon, D. A., and R. L. Phillips. "Coffee consumption and risk of fatal cancers." *American Journal of Public Health* 74, no. 8 (1984): 820–823.

Somchit, N., F. Sanat, E. H. Gan, A. W. Shahrin, and A. Zuraini. "Liver injury induced by the non-steroidal anti-inflammatory drug mefenamic acid." *Singapore Medical Journal* 45, no. 11 (2004): 530.

Spake, Amanda. *U.S. News and World Report*, Nov 8, 2004 [C. J. Gregor, "Acid suppression and pneumonia: A clinical indication for rational prescribing." *JAMA* 292 (2004): 2012–2013].

Steingraber, Sandra. "The Benefits of Breast Milk Outweigh Any Risks." CHEC's *HealtheHouse*, May 2002. www.checnet.org/healthehouse/education/articlesdetail. asp?Main_ID=451, May 2002.

Stephens, Francine. "Persistent Organic Pollutants: Chemicals That Won't Go Away and Hurt Us All." *Children's Health Environmental Coalition*, November 2002. www.checnet.org/healthehouse/education/articles-detail.asp?Main_ID=280.

Stone, Martin. "Lemon Balm," *Making Scents, Summer/Fall* 2004. From *Herbs Explained* by Martin Stone. Bloomington, IN: AuthorHouse, 2003.

Swan, S. H., R. L. Kruse, L. Fan, D. B. Barr, E. Z. Drobnis, J. B. Redmon, C. Wang, C. Brazil, J. W. Overstreet, and the Study for the Future of Families Research Group. "Semen quality in relation to biomarkers of pesticide exposure." *Environmental Health Perspectives* 111, no. 12 (2003): 1478–1484.

Talaly, P., and J. W. Fahey. "Phytochemicals from cruciferous plants protect against cancer by modulating carcinogen metabolism." *American Society for Nutritional Sciences Journal of Nutrition* 131 (November 2001): S3027–S3033.

Tavani, A., and C. La Vecchia. "Coffee, decaffeinated coffee, tea and cancer of the colon and rectum: A review of epidemiological studies, 1990–2003." *Cancer Causes and Control* 15, no. 8 (2004): 743–757.

Touchette, Nancy. "Pylori Paradox: Microbe Harms Stomach but Protects Esophagus." *Genome News Network*, April 4, 2003.

University of Pittsburgh Medical Center. "Irritable Bowel Syndrome: Treatment Options." http://irritablebowel.upmc.com/treatment.htm.

U.S. Food and Drug Administration. "Most recent warning letters." www.fda.gov.

———. Center for Devices and Radiological Health. www.fda.gov/cdrh.

Weiss, B., S. Amler, and R. W. Amler. "Pesticides." *Pediatrics* 113, no. 4 (2004): S1030–S1036. See full text at www.pediatrics.org.

Wholehealthmd.com. "Methionine: What is it?" www.wholehealthmd.com.

Wickner, Hali. "Cancer prevention, calcium and vitamin D." Dartmouth Medical School, January 12, 2004, study reported in *Journal of the National Cancer Institute*, December 3, 2003, www.dartmouth.edu/~vox/0304/0112/nutrients.html.

Wong, Cathy. "Arginine." www.about.com.

Woolcott, C. G., W. D. King, and L. D. Marrett. "Coffee and tea consumption and cancers of the bladder, colon and rectum." *European Journal of Cancer Prevention* 11, no. 2 (2002): 137–145.

Younglai, E. V., W. G. Foster, E. G. Hughes, K. Trim, and J. F. Jarrell. "Levels of environmental contaminants in human follicular fluid, serum, and seminal plasma of couples undergoing in vitro fertilization." *Archives of Environmental Contamination and Toxicology* 43, no. 1 (2002): 121–126.

Zeegers, M. P., F. E. Tan, R. A. Goldbohm, and P. A. van den Brandt. "Are coffee and tea consumption associated with urinary tract cancer risk? A systematic review and meta-analysis." *International Journal of Epidemiology* 30, no. 2 (2001): 353–362.

INDEX

floor exercises, 117–120
hatha yoga, 109
and irritable bowel syndrome, 71
and the lymphatic system, 53
and release of toxins, 14
sitting forward bend series,
120–123
standing exercises, 114–116
toilet exercises, 110–113
walking, 92–93, 110
weight maintenance, 85, 109
while fasting, 92–93

F

fasting. see also Weekend
Cleanse
bathing, 96–97
benefits, 93
dental care, 95–96
drink choices, 98–101
elimination of toxins, 88
juice fasting, 93–94, 100–101
laxatives, 97
and release of toxins, 14
side effects, 95, 103
supplements and medications, 97
who should not participate,
89, 94
fats
in modern diet, 17
and nutrition, 23–24
rancid, 43
fatty acids, 24, 43
fertility, 12
fiber
benefits, 18–23, 83–84
cancer prevention, 83–84
constipation prevention, 20, 64
and hunger satiation, 19
and irritable bowel syndrome,
70–71
in modern diet, 18–19
plant fiber illustration, 19

fluids
and digestion, 25–26
and fasting, 94, 99–100
food additives, 11
food intolerance, 70, 72
food sensitivity, 72
fried foods and liver function,
41, 43
fruit pectin, 45, 100
fruits and vegetables, 40, 83, 84

G

gallbladder, 44–45
gallstones, 45
garlic, 82
giardia infection, 74–75
glucose, 17–18
glutathione, 40–41
graham crackers, 21

H

healing process, 126–127
heartburn, 33, 35, 81
hemorrhoids, 20, 60, 63
hunger, feedback mechanisms,
16–17, 19
hydrogenated fats, 24
hyperventilation, 107

I

immune system, 37, 38, 72–73, 109
infants. see children
intestinal microflora
friendly bacteria, 43, 48, 50,
100
and leaky gut syndrome, 72
probiotics, 50, 51–52
irradiated foods, 50–51
irritable bowel syndrome (IBS),
20, 69–72

J

juice fasting, 93–94, 100–101

Simple Cleanse

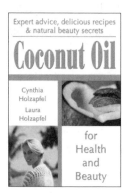
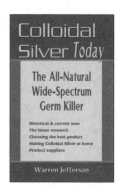
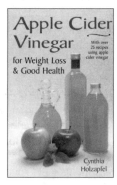
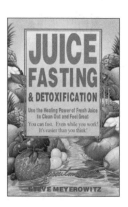
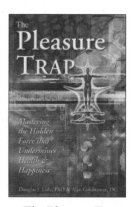
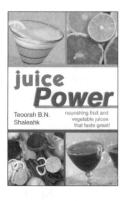